Making Sense of Critical Appraisal

To Ireti Oredola …

Making Sense of Critical Appraisal

O. Ajetunmobi MB BS MRCPsych
Specialist Registrar in General Psychiatry,
Towers Hospital, Leicester

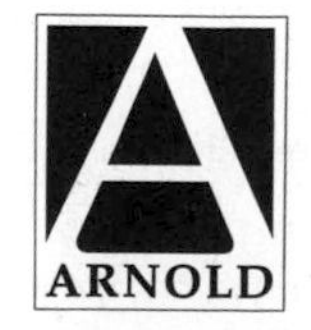

A member of the Hodder Headline Group
LONDON

First published in Great Britain in 2002 by
Arnold a member of the Hodder Headline Group,
338 Euston Road, London NW1 3BH

http://www.arnoldpublishers.com

Distributed in the USA by
Oxford University Press Inc.,
198 Madison Avenue, New York NY 10016
Oxford is a registered trademark of Oxford University Press

Whilst the advice and information in this book are believed to be true and accurate at the date of going to press, neither the author nor the publisher can accept any legal responsibility or liability for any errors or omissions that may be made. In particular (but without limiting the generality of the preceding disclaimer) every effort has been made to check drug dosages; however, it is still possible that errors have been missed. Furthermore, dosage schedules are constantly being revised and new side-effects recognized. For these reasons the reader is strongly urged to consult the drug companies' printed instructions before administering any of the drugs recommended in this book.

British Library Cataloguing in Publication Data
A catalogue record for this book is available from the British Library

Library of Congress Cataloging-in-Publication Data
A catalog record for this book is available from the Library of Congress

ISBN 0 340 80812 8 (pb)

1 2 3 4 5 6 7 8 9 10

Commissioning Editor: Georgina Bentliff
Development Editor: Heather Smith
Production Editor: Jasmine Brown
Production Controller: Bryan Eccleshall
Cover Design: Terry Griffiths

Typeset in 9/11 Palatino by Charon Tec Pvt. Ltd, Chennai, India
Printed and bound in Italy by Giunti

Contents

Introduction

In keeping with the ethos of evidence-based medical practice, critical appraisal of research papers has been introduced into the examination curricula of both undergraduate and postgraduate medical programmes alike. These new kinds of examinations are designed to test candidates' ability to critique the quality of evidence presented in research papers for clinical relevance.

Although many helpful courses and workshops do exist, it is a generally shared feeling among examinees and trainers alike that being a relatively new entity, the scope of critical appraisal as a subject remains somewhat unclear. To further muddy the waters, few concise texts geared towards examinations on critical appraisal exist to date, rendering exam preparation a tedious task in already unchartered territory. Unsurprisingly, therefore, some candidates approach this aspect of their examinations with an understandable degree of trepidation.

Ironically, once mastered, critical appraisal examinations represent an area in which candidates can score highly with a relatively high degree of certainty. This is less the case for essay or multiple-choice papers, never mind clinical examinations.

My intention in writing this book was to provide candidates with an easy-to-use exam-oriented text that covers most aspects of critical appraisal. Concepts are presented in a user-friendly format, particularly for the benefit of those who, like myself, find epidemiological and statistical concepts rather migraine-inducing.

Examinations apart, this book would also be a handy resource for all doctors and other professionals seeking to improve their skills at understanding and evaluating clinical research papers.

The first chapter deals with relevant aspects of general statistics and study design. This provides a solid basis for approaching the other chapters, which have been deliberately organized according to the types of studies that may be presented in research papers.

Chapters on economic analyses, qualitative research principles and clinical audit have been included, and the book also contains a glossary of epidemiological and statistical terms and definitions.

For the sake of clarity, fictitious research scenarios are presented alongside the main text where appropriate.

Enjoy!

Basic stats

1

Introduction

Critical appraisal is concerned with the acquisition of necessary skills with which to discern clinical research papers accurately. Although it is only natural that some degree of overlap does exist between the two subjects, critical appraisal should not really be regarded as just another aspect of medical statistics. This misconception often leads to an over-estimation of the level of statistical knowledge required for critical appraisal.

In this chapter, only the statistical concepts that are relevant to the purposes of critical appraisal are discussed. These concepts are carefully presented in a gentle step-by-step approach with aid of 'easily understandable' vignettes as necessary.

A separate 'Non-essential information' section is included for the more adventurous reader who may also want to consult more formal statistical texts for a more in-depth treatment of the various statistical concepts discussed.

Descriptive statistics

Types of data

Data can be described according to a variety of characteristics. Distinguishing between different types of data is a fundamental issue in statistics because it determines the way that data are handled and presented (Figure 1.1).

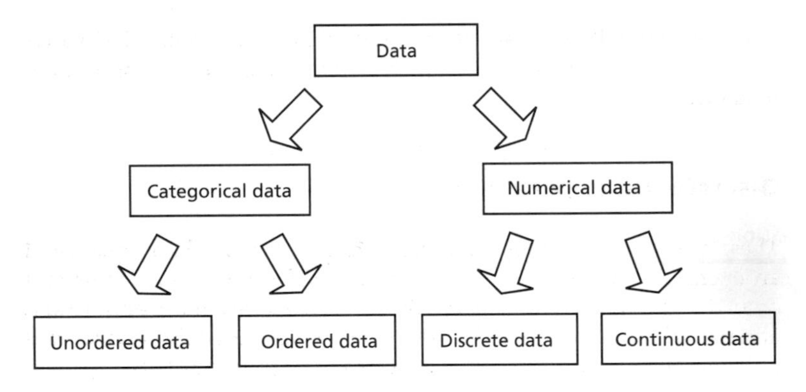

Figure 1.1 Classification of data.

Categorical data

These are qualitative data that cannot be measured on a scale and have no numerical value. Instead, they are identified, named and counted. The different types of categorical data can be described as follows:

- Nominal data (*binary*) – These can only be grouped into two categories. Examples include *either/or, dead/alive, improved/not improved, healed/unhealed, male/female observations,* etc.
- Nominal data (*multi-category*) – These can be grouped into more than two categories. Examples include racial groups, religious groups, social class, hair colour, television channels or questionnaire responses such as *'strongly disagree/disagree/don't know/agree/strongly agree'*, etc.
- Ranked data – These also have multiple categories but here, a hierarchy can be seen to exist between the respective categories. For example, following a head injury patients may be grouped into ranks of

mild, moderate and severe impairment; chemotherapy treatment response can be ranked as *'no response/partial response/partial remission/full remission'*, etc. Ranked categorical data are also called 'ordinal data'.

Ranked data can also be continuous in nature, for example visual analogue scale scores.

Numerical data

These are quantitative data, that is, data that have a numerical value. They can be further classified as being either 'discrete' or 'continuous' in nature.

Discrete numerical data

These are numerical data that exist as counts, that is, the frequency of an event. Examples include 'number of children' or 'number of cars owned', etc. These data can only take any of a discrete number of values and not values in between. Therefore, Mrs Smith cannot be said to have 3.67 children nor can her ex-husband be said to own 4.528 cars!

Continuous numerical data

This describes numerical data that can take any value within a given range. Examples of continuous data that can be gathered from a sample of people include age, body weight, height, temperature, time elapsed to an event, head circumference, etc.

Numerical data can also be subclassified in other ways but most of these are unimportant to the purposes of critical appraisal with the exception of the 'Normal distribution' and 'non-Normal distribution' classification. As will be seen later in this chapter, this is an important distinction that affects the way numerical data are regarded and handled in statistics.

Summarizing data

Describing data observations in such a way as to be universally understandable is the reason for summarizing data.

Consider the following responses obtained from a recently conducted survey of 20 postmen, regarding the number of dog attacks they had experienced whilst on their postal rounds over the preceding 10 years (Table 1.1).

Table 1.1 Responses obtained from a survey of 20 postmen

Postman	1	2	3	4	5	6	7	8	9	10	11	12	13	14	15	16	17	18	19	20
No. of attacks	4	6	2	6	7	1	50	0	0	4	5	2	4	1	6	1	3	2	1	0

Summarizing data involves the use of appropriate descriptive measures, most of which are already familiar to the reader. Ideally, the measures used in summarizing data should describe the centrality of data observations (*location*) as well as the diversity of data observations (*data spread*).

'Mean' and 'median' measures are used in describing data location (*central tendency*), whereas the 'standard deviation' (SD) and 'interquartile range' (IQR) measures are used in describing data spread (*lateral tendency*).

Although not a fixed rule, the mean and standard deviation are used together when describing 'normal' data, whereas the median and interquartile range are used together with 'skewed data'. Normal and skewed data are discussed in a later section.

Mean

The mean value of a data set can be determined simply by summing up all observations (Σx) and dividing this sum by the number of observations (n). From the postman data set, the mean number of dog attacks can be calculated by the formula:

$$\text{Mean } (\overline{x}) = \frac{\Sigma x}{n} = \frac{105}{20} = 5.25$$

The determination of a mean therefore involves the incorporation of the values of all observations in a data set. In other words, every data observation is used and this is a really nice thing about using the mean as a descriptive measure. However, using every data observation also renders the mean vulnerable to unusually large or unusually small observations, as seen with the unlucky Postman 7 in Table 1.1. Such eccentric observations are called 'outliers'. The mean is best used as a descriptive measure with data that obey a Normal distribution though it can also provide useful information with skewed data.

Table 1.2 Ranked responses from the survey of postmen

0	0	0	1	1	1	1	2	2	**2**	**3**	4	4	4	5	6	6	6	7	50

Median

The median represents the middle value of ordered data observations. If data were organized in an ascending or descending order, the value of the middle observation is said to be the 'median value'. In data sets with an even number of observations (such as with our postman data set), the median value can be determined by taking the mean of the middle two observations (Table 1.2).

$$\text{Median} = \frac{2+3}{2} = 2.5$$

As evident from the above example, a median value does not incorporate the values of all observations in its determination. Although this wastage of information is a weakness of the median measure, it also protects the median from outliers, therefore increasing the stability of the median as a descriptive measure. Generally, the median is used as a descriptive measure with skewed continuous data and even with discrete or categorical data.

Data variability

Consider that data were gathered on a million newborn babies regarding the number of normally formed digits at birth. Judging from the prevalence figures on congenital digit anomaly, these data are not likely to show much variability. In other words, an overwhelmingly large amount of data would have the same value.

Alternatively, consider that data were gathered on a million newborn babies regarding their birth weight. Judging from the documented figures on birth weight, these data are likely to show much more variability than would be seen with the digit anomaly data.

These different data sets illustrate the concept of 'data spread' and the need for a statistical measure that can describe such variability in a data set. As shown later on in this chapter, the degree of variability observed in a data set is an important factor that is taken into consideration when performing statistical analyses.

Standard deviation (SD)

The 'standard deviation' (SD) is a statistical measure that describes the extent of data spread or scatter. It is quoted alongside the mean to describe data spread where data is known to (at least approximately) obey a Normal distribution. The reader may wish to calculate the standard deviation for the postman data set by following the steps described below.

HOW TO CALCULATE A STANDARD DEVIATION (SD)

- SD is obtained by measuring the distance of each observation (x) from the mean ($\bar{x}$).

$$(\bar{x} - x)$$

- These respective distances are first squared and then added together.

$$\Sigma(\bar{x} - x)^2$$

- This sum is divided by the number of observations less one, to produce variance.

$$\frac{\Sigma(\bar{x} - x)^2}{n - 1}$$

- Finally, the square root of variance forms the standard deviation.

$$\text{SD} = \sqrt{\frac{\Sigma(\bar{x} - x)^2}{n - 1}}$$

(Answer: SD = 10.77.)

Interquartile range (IQR)

The 'interquartile range' (IQR) is a statistical measure describing the extent of spread of the middle 50% of ranked data. IQR is commonly used alongside a median value when describing the spread of skewed data. As illustrated below, three quartiles (lower, median and upper quartiles) are used to divide ranked data into four equal parts (Figure 1.2).

IQR is equivalent to the value of the upper quartile minus the value of the lower quartile (Table 1.3). Unlike standard deviation, IQR is not influenced by extreme values (*outliers*) and is relatively easy to calculate. However, IQR does not incorporate all presented observations, which is a weakness of this descriptive measure.

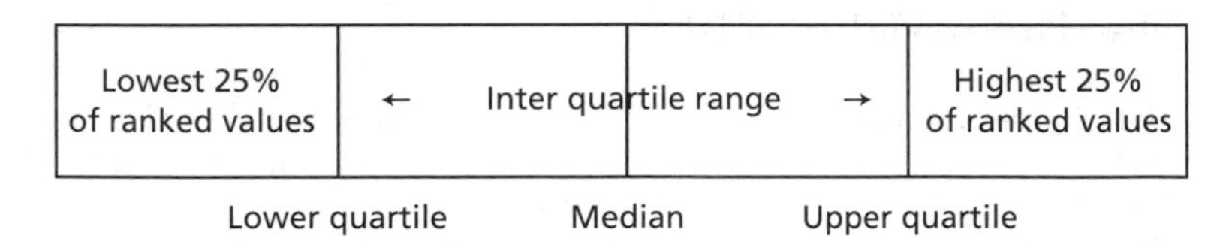

Figure 1.2 The interquartile range (IQR).

Table 1.3 IQR from the postman data set

0	0	0	1	1	1	1	2	2	2	3	4	4	4	5	6	6	6	7	50
					▲ Lower quartile									▲ Upper quartile					

Lower quartile = 1, that is, same value present on either side of the lower quartile. For the upper quartile, a weighted mean is taken between 5 and 6:

$$= \left(5 \times \frac{1}{4}\right) + \left(6 \times \frac{3}{4}\right) = 5.75$$

Interquartile range:

$$= 5.75 - 1 = 4.75.$$

In published papers, this interquartile range would usually be expressed as 'from 1 to 5.75'.

Normal distribution

In a Normal distribution (also known as 'Gaussian distribution'), observations with moderate values have higher frequencies, whereas those with more extreme values have lower frequencies. A Normal distribution therefore has a characteristic bell shape formed by a peak that slopes symmetrically downwards on either side. It is more often the case than not that numerical data obey a Normal distribution (Figure 1.3).

For example, the height data of adult men in a population would be likely to follow a Normal distribution. Moderate height values would be observed in the majority of adult men whilst a minority would be either very short or very tall men.

The mid-point (*median*) of a perfect Normal distribution also represents the mean value of the concerned parameter in the population.

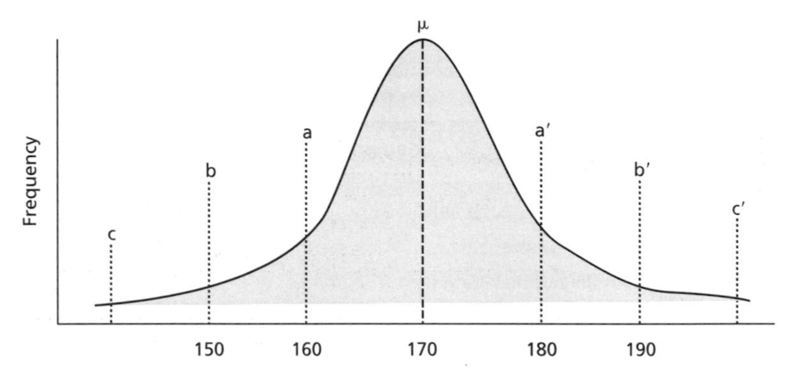

Figure 1.3 Normal distribution curve.

This is to be found in the centre of the plot denoted (μ). Therefore in a perfect Normal distribution the median value is equivalent to the mean value. The vertical lines denoted a, b and c (or a′, b′ and c′) represent approximately one, two and three standard deviations from the mean, respectively.

The real beauty of Normal distribution, however, is that it applies to such a large number of examples in medicine, although some types of data (e.g. time spent in hospital) can have differently shaped distributions. Standard deviation (SD), a measure of data spread, also has a number of very convenient properties within a Normal distribution. These convenient properties are described below.

In a Normal distribution:

- 68% of data observations will fall within the area between one standard deviation either side of the mean (i.e. a to a′).
- 95% of data observations will fall within the area between approximately two (1.96) standard deviations either side of the mean (i.e. b to b′).
- 99% of data observations will fall within the area between approximately three (2.58) standard deviations either side of the mean (c to c′).

Therefore, whenever data are known to (at least approximately) obey a Normal distribution, the above-described proportions of data falling into respective standard deviations can be taken for granted as being safe predictions (Figure 1.4).

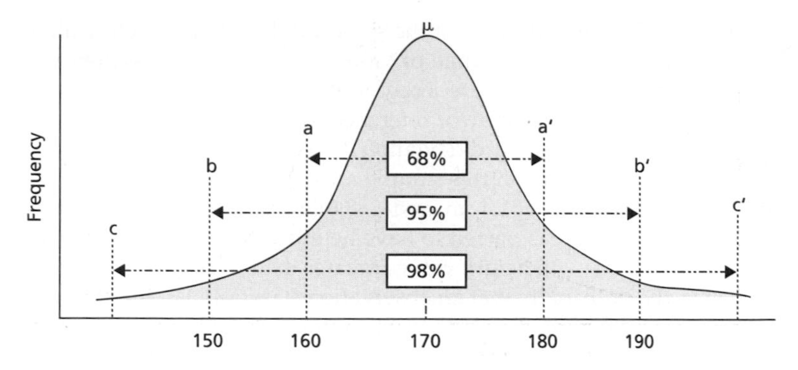

Figure 1.4 Standard deviation (SD) within a Normal distribution.

From population to sample

Measuring the heights of all adult men in an entire population is not practically possible in the real world. Therefore, in order to gain an insight into the adult male height distribution in a population, a *randomly selected* sample would need to be taken from that population.

Selection by a random process ensures that all members of the population would have had an equal chance of being chosen into the sample. This guarantees that the sample is indeed a truly representative window into the population.

EXAMPLE

Let us assume that 100 men are randomly selected from a population, and that from their height data, mean height is found to be 170 cm with a standard deviation (SD) of 9.5 cm. With these figures, the following predictions can be made about the sample (and therefore the entire population) from the Normal distribution: 95% of the sample would fall within 1.96 SDs either side of the mean (i.e. b to b′).

$$\begin{aligned} &\bar{x} - 1.96\,\text{SD to } \bar{x} + 1.96\,\text{SD} \\ &= 170 - (1.96 \times 9.5) \text{ to } 170 + (1.96 \times 9.5) \\ &= 151.4 \text{ to } 188.6\,\text{cm} \end{aligned}$$

In other words, 95% of the men in this sample will have height values between 151.4 cm and 188.6 cm!

These interesting attributes of the standard deviation therefore allow us to predict accurately a range of values within which specified proportions of the population are likely to be. These are called 'reference ranges' in statistics. As shown, reference ranges are derived from the mean value ($\overline{x}$) and standard deviation (SD) of a sample parameter.

Since 95% of the men in this sample are expected to have height values ranging between 151.4 cm and 188.6 cm, this leaves a remaining 2.5% of men who are expected to have height values less than 151.4 cm and another 2.5% with height values greater than 188.6 cm.

Hence, the probability that an observation (x) would fall further away from the sample mean than by 1.96 SDs either side of the mean is 5% or less. In other words, the probability that any of the men in the sample would actually be shorter than 151.4 cm or taller than 188.6 cm is 5% or less (i.e. $p = 0.05$).

Similarly:

- 99% of the sample would fall within 2.58 SDs either side of the mean (i.e. c to c').

$$\begin{aligned}&\overline{x} - 2.58\ \text{SD} \ \text{ to } \ \overline{x} + 2.58\ \text{SD}\\&\quad = 170 - (2.58 \times 9.5) \text{ to } 170 + (2.58 \times 9.5)\\&\quad = 145.5\ \text{cm to } 194.5\ \text{cm}\end{aligned}$$

In other words, 95% of the men in this sample will have height values between 145.5 cm and 194.5 cm!

Therefore, 99% of the men in this sample are expected to have height values ranging between 145.5 cm and 194.5 cm. This leaves a remaining 0.5% of men who are expected to have height values less than 145.5 cm and another 0.5% of men with height values greater than 194.5 cm.

Hence, the probability that an observation (x) would fall further away from the sample mean than by 2.58 SDs either side of the mean is 1% or less. In other words, the probability that any of the men in the sample would actually be shorter than 145.5 cm or taller than 194.5 cm is 1% or less ($p = 0.01$).

In fact, the probability associated with obtaining any given observation (x) in a Normal distribution can be determined in this way, by measuring the distance of the observation from the sample mean, that is:

$$(\overline{x} - x)$$

then determining how many SDs from the mean this distance represents, that is:

$$\frac{(\overline{x} - x)}{\text{SD}}$$

and then working out the probability of getting such an observation so far away from the mean value using a pre-prepared z-distribution table such as Table i (see 'Non-essential information' at the end of this chapter).

EXAMPLE 1

What is the probability that a man selected from the sample population would be 183 cm tall? (Sample mean ($\bar{x}$) = 170 cm; SD = 9.5 cm.)

Distance of observation from sample mean ($\bar{x} - x$):

$$= 170 - 183\,\text{cm} = 13\,\text{cm}$$

That is, disregard negative sign as we are only interested in knowing that (x) is 13 cm away from ($\bar{x}$). 1.37 SD is called a 'z statistic'. From Table i, $z = 1.37$ SD corresponds to a probability of 0.16. Denoted as $p = 0.17$.

EXAMPLE 2

What is the probability that a man selected from the sample population would be 140 cm tall? (Sample mean ($\bar{x}$) = 170 cm; SD = 9.5 cm.)

Distance of observation from sample mean ($\bar{x} - x$):

$$= 170 - 140\,\text{cm} = 30\,\text{cm}$$

That is, (x) is 30 cm away from ($\bar{x}$). This distance of 30 cm represents 3.16 SD (30/9.5) away from sample mean ($\bar{x}$). 3.16 SD is called a 'z statistic'. From Table i, $z = 3.16$ SD corresponds to a probability less than 0.0020. Denoted as $p < 0.002$.

Hypothesis testing and statistical inference

In contrast to the previous section in which descriptive measures and their properties within a single population were explored, this section is concerned with comparing different populations (samples) for a difference regarding a specific parameter, for example mean values.

The null hypothesis (H?)

The null hypothesis states that 'No relationship exists between the variable(s) and outcome of a study'. The null hypothesis is the primary assumption on which statistical calculations are based. It is a statement of *non-association* and is regarded as the presumed answer to any scientific question, until proved otherwise. The implication of this non-association stance of the null hypothesis is that any observed associations occur by pure chance.

Research question:	Does cigarette smoking cause lung cancer?
Null hypothesis:	Cigarette smoking does not cause lung cancer.
Alternative hypothesis:	Cigarette smoking causes lung cancer.
Research question:	Does a relationship exist between alcoholism and suicide?
Null hypothesis:	No relationship exists between alcoholism and suicide.
Alternative hypothesis:	A relationship does exist between alcoholism and suicide.

The 'alternative hypothesis' is the proposed experimental hypothesis that invariably runs contrary to the null hypothesis in a study. However, when contemplating a research question, a scientist must start with the presumption that the null hypothesis actually holds true in that instance. An experiment is then devised in order to test this non-association prediction, that is, hypothesis testing.

Type I error

A Type I error is also known as an 'α-error'. In an experiment, a Type I error is said to occur if the null hypothesis is *rejected* when it is actually true. In other words, to find a significant difference between samples when really, none exists!

Significance testing is the safety mechanism that guards against wrongful rejection of the null hypothesis (Type I error) in a study, a process that involves quoting associated *p*-values alongside result findings.

p-values

'*P*-values' are probability figures that express the chance of obtaining a given result, in light of a true null hypothesis. They are used in deciding whether to accept or reject the null hypothesis in a study. Significant results are those that are statistically deemed as being unlikely to have occurred by chance thus rejecting the null hypothesis, whereas non-significant results are those in which a chance occurrence has not been ruled out, that is, the null hypothesis has not been disproved.

If the null hypothesis were true:

- $p < 0.5$ means the probability of obtaining a given result by chance is less than one in two.
- $p < 0.1$ means the probability of obtaining a given result by chance is less than one in 10.
- $p < 0.05$ means the probability of obtaining a given result by chance is less than one in 20.
- $p < 0.025$ means the probability of obtaining a given result by chance is less than one in 40.
- $p < 0.01$ means the probability of obtaining a given result by chance is less than one in 100.

By a totally arbitrary convention, '$p < 0.05$' is the accepted threshold for statistical significance. In other words, $p < 0.05$ represents the minimum degree of evidence needed in order to discard the null hypothesis. p-values greater than 0.05 are deemed non-significant, whereas p-values less than 0.05 are deemed statistically significant (Table 1.4).

Table 1.4 Relationship between p-values*, significance and the null hypothesis

If $p < 0.05$ quoted with results	Probability result occurred by chance is less than 1 in 20	Results deemed significant	Null hypothesis judged false and is rejected	Evidence of association between variable and outcome accepted
If $p > 0.05$ quoted with results	Probability result occurred by chance is greater than 1 in 20	Results deemed non-significant	Null hypothesis cannot be rejected	Association between variable and outcome unproven

* p-values express the probability of getting observed results given a true null hypothesis.

How *p*-values are actually calculated

In order to calculate a p-value, a statistical test is used to compare the values of a parameter (e.g. mean height values) obtained from two different populations. To illustrate how such a comparison is made, we need to extend our 'male height' vignette to compare height values between two different populations of adult men... say right and left handed men respectively.

We do this by gathering two sets of data, one from 100 right-handed men and another from 100 left-handed men all randomly selected from their respective populations.

Naming our right-handed sample 'Sample a' and left-handed sample 'Sample b', a comparison may be made between both, regarding differences in mean height by applying a *z*-test (only used for very large samples) as described below.

Note that a *z*-test is used when making comparisons between continuous data gathered from two large samples. For smaller sized samples, (i.e. samples with approximately less than 30 observations), the '*t*-test' is used instead. Get a formal stats book if you really need to know why!

z-TEST: EXAMPLE 1

Imagine that the mean and standard deviation (SD) quoted for Sample a was 170 cm and 9.5 cm and for Sample b was 160 cm and 13 cm, respectively. Regarding the height, how different are samples a and b?

Null hypothesis

Subjects in both samples belong to the same population and no real height differences exist between them (i.e. a = b).

Alternative hypothesis

Subjects in the compared samples are too dissimilar to have come from the same population (i.e. a ≠ b).

Comparing means

What is the probability of obtaining such discrepant mean height values if all subjects were really from the same population?

Sample a	Sample b
Mean height ($\bar{x}$a) = 170 cm	Mean height ($\bar{x}$b) = 160 cm
Standard deviation (SDa) = 9.5 cm	Standard deviation (SDb) = 13 cm
Number in sample (*n*a) = 100	Number in sample (*n*b) = 100
Difference between sample means ($\bar{x}$b − $\bar{x}$a) = 10 cm	

The formula for calculating the standard error of the mean (SEM) difference between two samples:

$$\sqrt{\frac{\text{SDa}^2}{n\text{a}} + \frac{\text{SDb}^2}{n\text{b}}}$$

Standard error of mean difference:

$$\sqrt{0.90 + 1.69} = 1.61$$

Therefore, the z statistic, that is, how many standard errors is the mean difference:

$$= 10\,\text{cm}/1.61$$
$$z = 6.21$$

From Table i, $z = 6.21$ corresponds to a probability (p-value) of much less than 0.001 (i.e. $p < 0.001$).

Conclusion

If both sets of subjects really belonged to the same population and no real difference existed between them regarding height, the probability of obtaining results as discrepant as observed is less than one in 1000 ($p < 0.001$) and therefore the null hypothesis is rejected!

A 95% confidence interval (95% CI) can be determined for this mean difference of 4 cm between both samples according to the formula:

$$95\%\ \text{CI} = 10 \pm (1.91 \times 1.61) = 7.42\,\text{cm to } 12.58\,\text{cm}$$

In other words, if from the two respective populations, samples were repeatedly drawn and compared with each other, the difference in mean height values between each compared pair of samples would vary between 7.42 cm and 12.58 cm 95% of the time.

z-TEST: EXAMPLE 2

Now, imagine that the mean and standard deviation (SD) quoted for Sample b was 172 cm and 13 cm, respectively. Now, how different are samples a and b?

Null hypothesis

Subjects in both samples belong to the same population and no real height differences exist between them (i.e. a = b).

Alternative hypothesis

Subjects in the compared samples are too dissimilar to have come from the same population (i.e. a $\neq$ b).

Comparing means

What is the probability of obtaining such discrepant mean height values if all subjects were really from the same population?

Sample a	Sample b
Mean height ($\bar{x}$a) = 170 cm	Mean height ($\bar{x}$b) = 172 cm
Standard deviation (SDa) = 9.5 cm	Standard deviation (SDb) = 13 cm
Number in sample (*n*a) = 100	Number in sample (*n*b) = 100
Difference between sample means ($\bar{x}$b − $\bar{x}$a) = 2 cm	

The special standard error formula:

$$\sqrt{\frac{\text{SDa}^2}{na} + \frac{\text{SDb}^2}{nb}} = \sqrt{0.90 + 1.69} = 1.61$$

Therefore, the z statistic, that is, how many standard errors is the mean difference:

$$= 2\,\text{cm}/1.6$$
$$z = 1.24$$

From Table i, $z = 1.24$ corresponds to a probability (p-value) of $p < 0.2$.

Conclusion

If both sets of subjects were really from the same population and no real height differences existed between them, the probability of obtaining results as discrepant as observed is less than one in five ($p < 0.2$) and therefore the null hypothesis cannot be rejected!

A 95% confidence interval (95% CI) can be determined for this mean difference of 1 cm between both samples according to the formula:

$$95\%\ \text{CI} = 2 \pm (1.96 \times 1.61) = -0.58\,\text{cm to } 4.58\,\text{cm}$$

In other words, if from the two respective populations, samples were repeatedly drawn and compared with each other, the difference in mean height values between each compared pair of samples would vary between −0.58 cm and 4.58 cm 95% of the time. This range includes zero and therefore implies a non-significant difference.

One-tailed and two-tailed significance tests

In hypothesis testing (i.e. of the null hypothesis), significance tests may be used to examine only one direction of the alternative hypothesis,

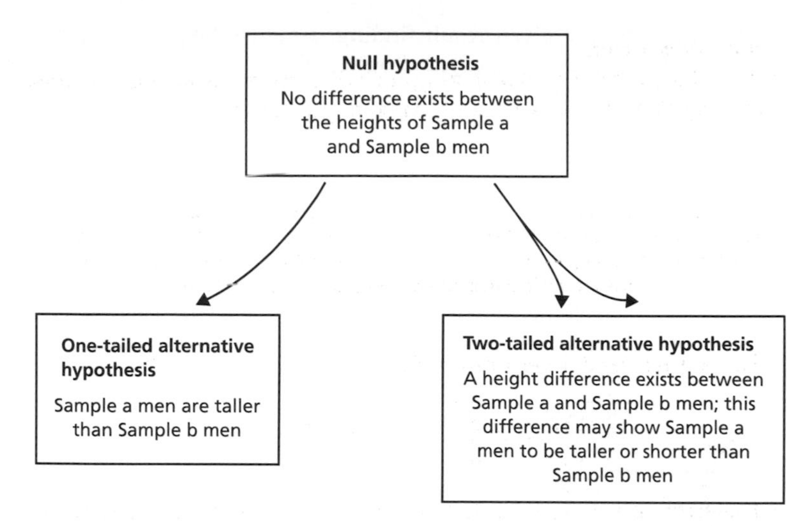

Figure 1.5 Examples of one-tailed and two-tailed testing.

disregarding the opposite direction. These are called 'one-tailed significance tests'. Alternatively, significance tests may make no assumptions about the direction of difference (examining both directions). These are 'two-tailed significance tests'.

One-tailed tests are less desirable than two-tailed tests and should only be used in situations where one of the directions of difference has been proved to be implausible (Figure 1.5).

Why test for significance?

By pure chance, even a chimpanzee can answer a difficult 'true or false' question item correctly with a one in two (0.5) probability. However, it is unlikely that such a correct response would envoke much excitement because a one in two probability is, frankly, not very convincing.

On the other hand, if our chimpanzee were able to select a correct response from among 99 other false responses, that is, a one in 100 (0.01) probability, it would be a circus star! Although this display of knowledge could similarly have resulted by pure chance, a one in 100 probability is much more convincing than the former scenario. This is much less likely to have been a fluke.

This 'simian' example illustrates the need for the use of *p*-values when presenting results. By conveying a sense of the fluke-factor associated with any given result finding, *p*-values help us to decide when and when not to get excited about results.

Type II error

A Type II error is also known as a 'β-error'. It is said to occur if the null hypothesis is *accepted* when it is actually false. In other words, failing to find a significant difference between samples when one really exists! The degree to which this folly is guarded against in a study is called the 'power' of that study.

Power

The power of a study is defined as the probability that a Type II error will not be made in that study. As a general rule, the larger the sample size of a study the more *power* the study is said to have (i.e. the probability that a significant difference will be found … if one really existed). Therefore, a calculation is necessary before the start of a study to determine how large the sample size needs to be in order to achieve the degree of power chosen for that study. For example, a power of 0.9 means you have 90% probability of finding a significant difference with a given sample size, if a real difference truly did exist, having excluded the role of chance.

By arbitrary convention, a power of 0.8 is generally accepted as being adequate in most research studies. Still, the power of a study can be enhanced by other methodological factors other than sample size. These are factors that further increase the chance of finding the truth with any given sample size, for example using more precise measuring instruments.

WHO PERFORMS A SAMPLE SIZE CALCULATION?

Thankfully, only statisticians or other competent professionals should carry out this task. Study reports should describe their sample size calculations in detail.

SAMPLE SIZE CALCULATIONS

These are carried out before the start of a study so as to determine the sample size that would be necessary for the required power in that particular study. A sample size caculation takes several factors into account. These include:

- The number of different properties being considered.
- The number of groups being compared.
- The variability of property being measured.
- An estimate of proposed difference between compared groups (smallest true mean difference that would be clinically viable).
- The significance level required (how much proof?).
- The degree of power required (how much vigilance?).

Sample size formula:

$$n \geqslant \frac{2\sigma^2(\varepsilon_{\alpha/2} + \varepsilon_{\beta})^2}{\delta^2}$$

n = number of subjects required in each group;
σ = standard deviation of property;
α = significance level (e.g. if $\sigma = 0.05$ then $\alpha/2 = 0.025$ and $\alpha/2 = 1.96$);
$\beta = 1 -$ power (e.g. if power $= 0.9$ then $\beta = 0.1$ and $\beta = 1.282$);
δ = estimated size of difference or effect.

Example: consider a study interested in proving that right-handed men are, on the whole, taller than left-handed men. The necessary sample size calculation would have to take the following factors into consideration:

- Number of properties being considered = one (height).
- Number of groups being compared = two groups (right- and left-handed men).
- Degree of height variability (height standard deviation).
- An estimate of the proposed height difference between both groups.
- The required significance test (e.g. $p < 0.05$).
- The required power (e.g. 0.8).

Estimation

Discussion so far has been on descriptive measures as they apply to a sample whose data obey the Normal distribution. However, we should remember that the mean value ($\bar{x}$) of a parameter obtained from one sample is only an estimation of the 'true' mean value (μ) of that parameter in the general population.

In fact, deriving the true mean value (μ) of a property in a population can be an almost-impossible task and may involve gathering data from an impossibly large or even an infinite number of repeated random samples. Even then, the respective mean values ($\overline{x}$) so obtained are likely to vary from sample to sample, with only an anonymous few actually corresponding to the true mean value (μ).

This variability of such repeated sample means is influenced by two principal factors:

- The greater the baseline variability of a property in the general population (i.e. the standard deviation), the more variability we would expect in the respective sample means ($\overline{x}$) derived from repeated samples.
- The larger the size of respective samples, the less variability we would expect in derived sample means.

Standard error (SE)

The above-described variability that would occur from sample to sample when estimating the value of a parameter is expressed by a statistical measure called the 'standard error' (SE) (Figure 1.6); in this case, the standard error of a mean value (SEM). Stated differently, the standard error of a mean (SEM) can be said to express the likelihood of difference between a sample mean ($\overline{x}$) and the true mean value (μ) of a parameter in the general population.

The difficulty with determining the true value (μ) of a property is therefore overcome in statistics by expressing the likelihood of error associated with its estimate ($\overline{x}$). As already stated, factors which influence the

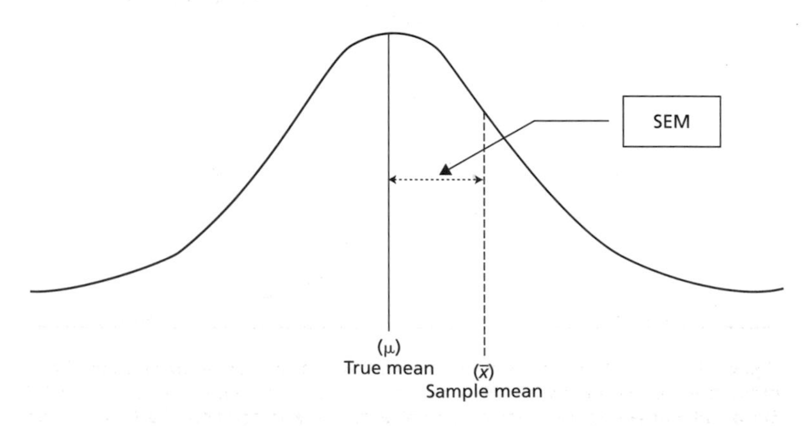

Figure 1.6 Standard error (SE) and formula.

SEM include the baseline variability of the measured property in the population (SD) and sample size (n). In fact, the formula:

$$\text{SEM} = \frac{\text{SD}}{\sqrt{n}}$$

Standard error should not be confused with standard deviation. SEM expresses the degree of uncertainty surrounding the mean value, whereas standard deviation simply reflects the degree of data variability about the mean value.

To summarize briefly, once we have estimated the true mean value (μ) of a property in the general population by deriving a mean value ($\bar{x}$) from a randomly selected sample, we know that there will have been some random error associated with our estimate ($\bar{x}$). This random error is expressed by the standard error measure.

Interestingly, if random samples were repeatedly taken from the same concerned population, and the derived mean values ($\bar{x}$) obtained from these repeated samples were presented on a plot; they would also obey a Normal distribution and be subject to the already-discussed features of a Normal distribution (Figure 1.7).

Using the Sample a data, mean height = 170 cm and standard error = 0.95(SD/n), the following assumptions can be safely made from the Normal distribution regarding the true mean value (μ) of a property in the general population: 95% of repeatedly derived mean values ($\bar{x}$) would fall in the area between 1.96 standard errors (i.e. B to B′) either side of the mean.

$$\begin{aligned}&(\bar{x} - 1.96\ \text{SE to } \bar{x} + 1.96\ \text{SE})\\ &\quad = 170 - (1.96 \times 0.95) \text{ to } 170 + (1.96 \times 0.95)\\ &\quad = 168.1\ \text{cm to } 171.9\ \text{cm}\end{aligned}$$

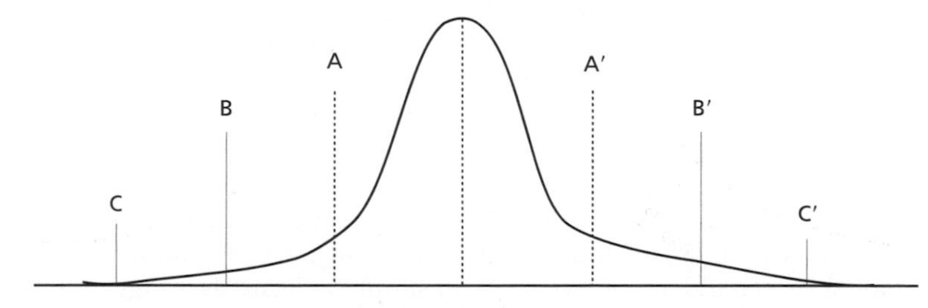

Figure 1.7 Standard error (SE) within a Normal distribution. Normal distribution plot of successive sample mean values ($\bar{x}$) and *not* of individual observations (x), as in Figure 1.7. Being a plot of sample mean values and not of raw data observations the SE (A, B, C or A′, B′, C′) becomes applicable instead of standard deviation (SD) (a, b, c or a′, b′, c′).

In other words, if several smaller samples were studied, 95% of all such derived mean values would fall between 168.1 cm and 171.9 cm! This range is called a 95% confidence interval!

In other words we can be 95% confident that the true mean height value (μ) lies somewhere between 168.1 cm and 171.9 cm.

Similarly, 99% of repeatedly derived mean values ($\bar{x}$) would fall in the area between 2.58 standard errors (i.e. C to C′) either side of the mean.

$$(\bar{x} - 2.58 \text{ SE to } \bar{x} + 2.58 \text{ SE})$$
$$= 170 - (2.58 \times 0.95) \text{ to } 170 + (2.58 \times 0.95)$$
$$= 167.5 \text{ cm to } 177.5 \text{ cm}$$

In other words, if several similar samples were studied, 99% of all such derived mean values would fall between 167.5 cm and 177.5 cm! This range is called a 99% confidence interval!

In other words we can be 99% confident that the true mean height value (μ) lies somewhere between 167.5 cm and 177.5 cm.

Confidence intervals

As already discussed (see 'Standard error' above), no one can be absolutely certain of an estimate. For example, if the sleep duration of 1000 people were measured in a study aiming to estimate 'the mean nocturnal sleep duration in Copenhagen', results would vary from person to person. However, somewhere among those varied results would be the *true* answer.

Short of actually timing the sleep duration of everybody in Copenhagen, the *true* mean value can only be estimated by taking an average of the responses obtained from smaller population samples. Even then, results would still vary from sample to sample.

It is an inescapable reality of life, therefore, that the making of estimates is always linked with a degree of uncertainty. In statistics, the degree of uncertainty surrounding an estimate can be expressed with use of confidence intervals. A confidence interval can therefore be defined as a range of values which, when quoted in relation to an estimate, express the degree of uncertainty around that estimate.

Hence if the mean sleep duration in Copenhagen is quoted at, say, 330 minutes with a 95% confidence interval of, say, 270–390 minutes, this quoted 95% confidence interval would simply indicate the range within which the true mean sleep duration is likely to be, with a 95% level of certainty.

In other words, if successive samples were randomly selected from the Copenhagen population, the respective mean values derived from these samples would lie within the stated confidence interval in 95% of attempts. Such is the essence and simplicity of confidence intervals that:

- 95% confidence intervals can be calculated according to the formula

$$95\%\ \text{CI} = \bar{x} \pm (1.96 \times \text{SE}).$$

- 99% confidence intervals can be calculated according to the formula

$$99\%\ \text{CI} = \bar{x} \pm (2.58 \times \text{SE}).$$

The tongue-in-cheek illustration below shows how we all use confidence interval principles in everyday life.

Peter:	How long is this train journey?
Mary:	Usually about one hour ... give or take five minutes. (Estimate 60 minutes; range 55–65 minutes.)
Peter:	I have to plan my journey to a job interview ... how sure are you?
Mary:	Well, I am 95% sure.
Peter:	What do you mean 95% sure?
Mary:	What I mean is that if you randomly selected and timed 100 journeys of this train, 95 of those 100 journeys would be between 55 and 65 minutes in duration. (Estimate 60 minutes; range 55–65 minutes.)
Peter:	I see, but it is imperative that I arrive on time for the interview! Could you not be 99% sure? What about the other five journeys?
Mary:	Well, of those five unusual journeys, some would be shorter than 55 minutes and others would be longer than 65 minutes. Hence, if I asked to be 99% sure, I would have to say that this train journey usually takes about one hour ... give or take 10 minutes. (Estimate 60 minutes; range 50–70 minutes.)
Peter:	Thank you Mary, you are so kind and so very clever.
Mary:	Cheers, fancy a drink?

Although technically not confidence intervals, the ranges quoted by Mary are nevertheless useful in understanding how the range of a confidence interval can be made wider or narrower by changes in any of the following factors.

a. The degree of confidence quoted

The example above demonstrates this clearly. The quoted '95% range' is narrower than the '99% range' quoted for the estimated journey time. Similarly, a confidence interval becomes wider in range as the degree of confidence increases. In other words, the higher the degree of confidence the wider the confidence interval would be.

b. Sample size

If 1000 randomly selected similar train journeys were timed as above instead of just 100, Mary would have been able to quote even narrower 95% and 99% ranges. This is because with 900 more train timings (*events*), she would be even surer of her facts.

c. Data variability

Going along with the above example, Mary would be more confident about giving narrower ranges at both 95% and 99% if only one train and one driver was involved in all the journeys than if several trains with several drivers took the journeys in turn. This is because increased data variability brings about increased unpredictability.

CONFIDENCE INTERVALS AND STATISTICAL SIGNIFICANCE

When quoted alongside a difference between two groups (e.g. mean difference), a confidence interval that includes zero is statistically non-significant.

When quoted alongside a ratio (e.g. relative risk, odds-ratio, etc.), a confidence interval that includes one is statistically non-significant.

WHY CONFIDENCE INTERVALS?

As 'proof statements', confidence intervals are increasingly preferred to the traditional *p*-values when presenting clinical results. This is mainly because even the smallest, most clinically inconsequential difference between compared groups can actually be statistically significant. This weakness associated with *p*-values is clinically unhelpful.

In other words, *p*-values can only tell us if a result observation is significant or not… and nothing more. All they can do is to express the strength of evidence against the null hypothesis. *P*-values are therefore limited in this dichotomy of 'significant versus non-significant'.

Furthermore, even the '$p < 0.05$' level at which results are deemed significant or non-significant is completely arbitrary, based on nothing more than a mere consensus among statisticians. Consensus on significance might have just as well been based on a '$p < 0.04$' level or a '$p < 0.03$' level.

Confidence intervals, on the other hand, are far more straightforward as proof statements and, as such, are much easier to relate to. Presented in the format of a range, they offer more information about the properties of a result observation at a glance *vis-à-vis* the magnitude, the clinical importance, the statistical significance, the (im)precision and a plausible range of the result finding. These advantages are illustrated in the example below.

Example

Some intuitive statisticians suspect that psychiatrists are generally better-looking than their other medical colleagues. They decide to set up a study comparing photographs of 100 psychiatrists with those of 100 doctors from other disciplines. All the photographs were randomly selected from the Medical Council photo register. In this study, the newly validated 'facial-assessment-scanner' that scores on a scale of 1–20 was used. The results are as follows:

- Psychiatrists: mean score 17; $n = 100$.
- Others: mean score 15; $n = 100$.
- Difference in means: 2 ($p < 0.01$; 95% CI 1.45–2.55).

All *p*-values can say about these results ($p < 0.01$) is: the difference found between psychiatrists and their other medical colleagues regarding looks is a significant one (i.e. $p < 0.01$). In other words, it is unlikely that this observed difference simply occurred by chance. If the null hypothesis were really true, such a chance result can only have happened in less than one in 100 cases and therefore we accept that this is a statistically significant finding.

What confidence intervals can say about these results (mean = 2; 95% CI 1.45–2.55):

- On average, psychiatrists score two points higher than their colleagues. This is the 'magnitude' of difference.
- This finding is statistically significant because the confidence intervals (95% CI 1.45–2.55) does not include zero.
- Furthermore, we have a 'plausible range' of difference regarding looks between the parties concerned because the observed difference of two points might vary between 1.45 and 2.55 in 95% of similar experiments.
- Inspecting the result and confidence interval allows us to judge the 'clinical importance' of the result findings.
- The plausible range also gives us an idea of the extent of '(im)precision' surrounding our estimate of a 'better-looking' effect direction.

Ideally, confidence intervals should be quoted along with appropriate *p*-values when presenting results.

Statistical tests

As a logical follow-on from the previous section, we now explore the different statistical tests that are employed in the calculation of the *p*-values and confidence intervals already described, and therefore, the statistical significance of data observations.

As medics employ cardiac enzymes in detecting cardiac pathology, liver enzymes for hepatic pathology, etc., so statisticians employ appropriate statistical tests in the analyses of different types of data. It is important that the appropriate statistical tests are used in the analyses of the different types of data so as to avoid grossly misleading *p*-values or confidence intervals that can result in erroneous judgements on significance.

From a critical appraisal standpoint, the main considerations when choosing which statistical tests to apply to data are:

- Categorical versus numerical data.
- Continuous versus non-continuous data.
- Unpaired versus paired data.

Categorical data

These are qualitative data that cannot be measured on a scale and have no numerical value. Instead, they are identified, named and counted. The different types of categorical data have already been discussed in a previous section and include nominal and ranked data.

Importantly, numerical data can often be converted into a ranked categorical format by applying cut-off points to the numerical values. This is usually done in order to increase the clinical relevance of numerical data. For example, using cut-off points, numerical data on body mass index gathered from a sample of patients can be converted into a ranked categorical format of *obese/overweight/normal/underweight/grossly underweight*. Clearly, a categorical format such as this would convey more meaningful information to patients and clinicians than a raw set of numbers.

Furthermore, the conversion of numerical data to a categorical format is also performed in order to render such data much easier to analyse. This is because categorical statistical tests are relatively simple to perform and involve the use of contingency tables (see below). However, when numerical data are analysed in this way, statistical power may be much reduced and the whole process becomes more Type II error-prone. Figure 1.8 describes the various statistical tests used with categorical data and their respective indications.

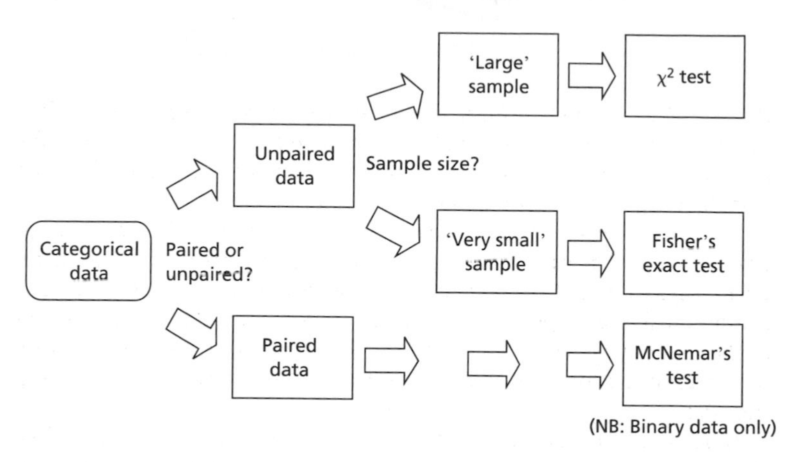

Figure 1.8 Categorical data statistical test flow chart.

The statistical tests used with categorical data are the 'chi-square' (χ^2) test (unpaired categorical data) and the 'McNemar's test' (paired binary data). A limitation with the chi-square test is that it can only provide approximate results. This limitation is however not really a problem with large-sized samples. For small-sized samples, however, (i.e. <5 observations in any cell), the 'Fisher's exact test' is a more appropriate instrument.

Contingency tables

In order to analyse categorical data, data are first cross-tabulated onto a contingency table consisting of rows and columns of cells in which respective events frequencies are recorded. Cross-tabulation is often used in presenting categorical data obtained from studies on diagnostic tests, cross-sectional surveys, case-control studies, prospective studies or randomized clinical trials (Figure 1.9).

Note that only frequencies can be entered into a contingency table. Other values such as percentages, proportions, averages, ratios or transformed values cannot and should not be cross-tabulated!

Continuous data

The main considerations when choosing which statistical tests to apply to continuous data are whether data are known to obey a Normal

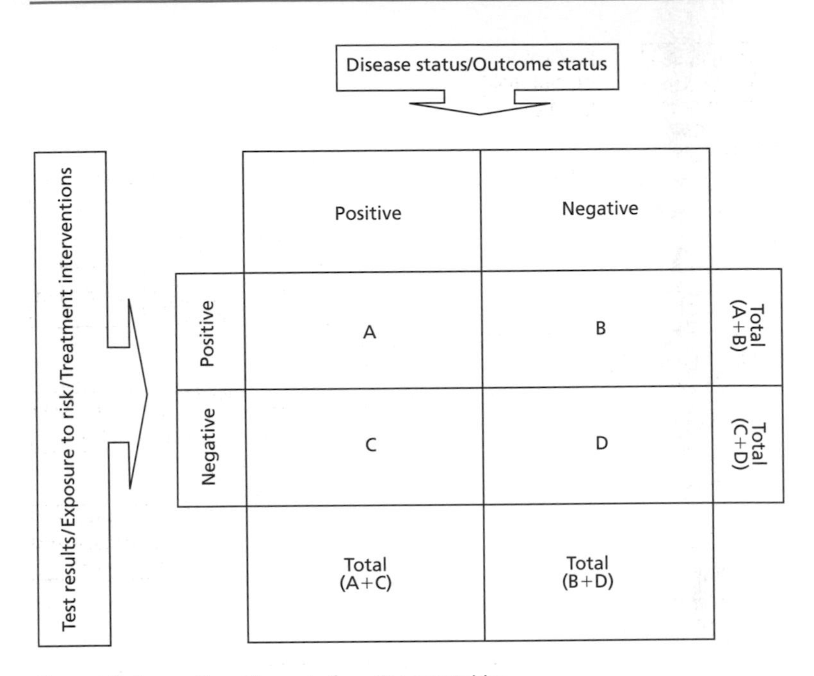

Figure 1.9 Conventional format of contingency tables.

distribution and whether any pairing is seen to exist in the data. Figure 1.10 describes the various statistical tests used with continuous data and their respective indications.

Normal data and parametric statistical tests

As already discussed, conveniently in a Normal distribution, 68% of observations lie in the area between one standard deviation either side of the mean (a to a′). Furthermore, 95% of observations lie within the area between approximately two standard deviations (b to b′) and 99% of observations between approximately three standard deviations either side of the mean (c to c′).

These interesting properties of the Normal distribution are a few of the many assumptions that parametric statistical tests make when used in statistical calculations. Parametric tests should be used whenever data are known to at least approximately obey a Normal distribution. They are more powerful than the non-parametric tests. The parametric

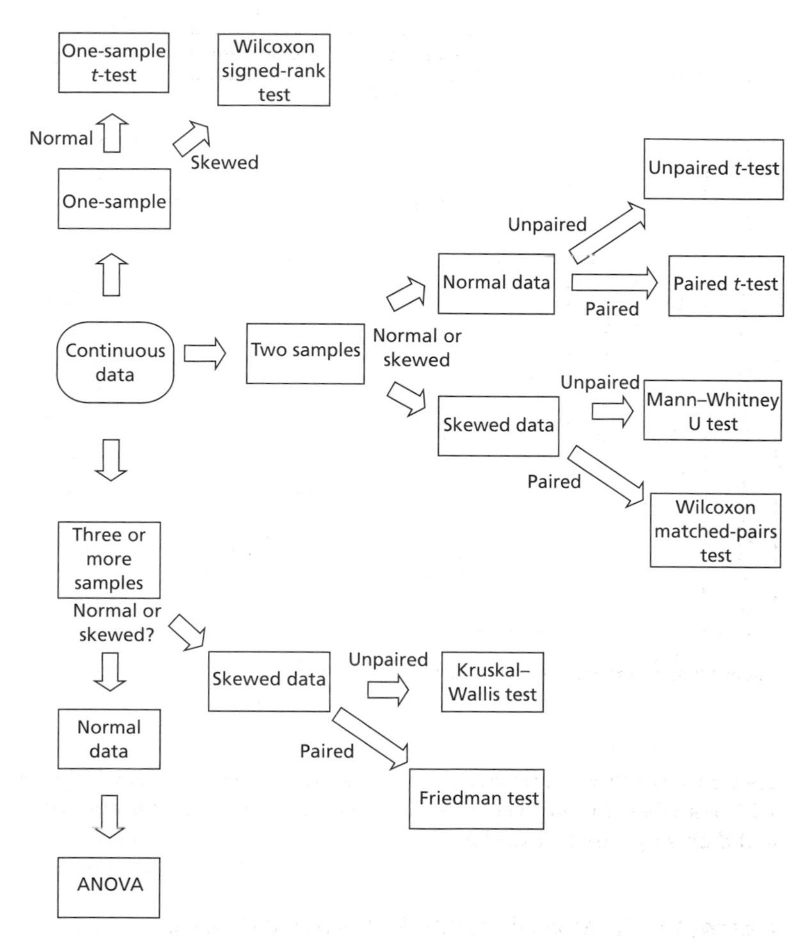

Figure 1.10 Continous data statistical test flow chart.

tests used when comparing continuous data from two groups are the 'unpaired *t*-test' (*unpaired data*) and the 'paired *t*-test' (*paired data*).

Skewed data and non-parametric tests

Very often, and particularly with small samples, continuous data may not obey a Normal distribution. In such situations, skewed data can

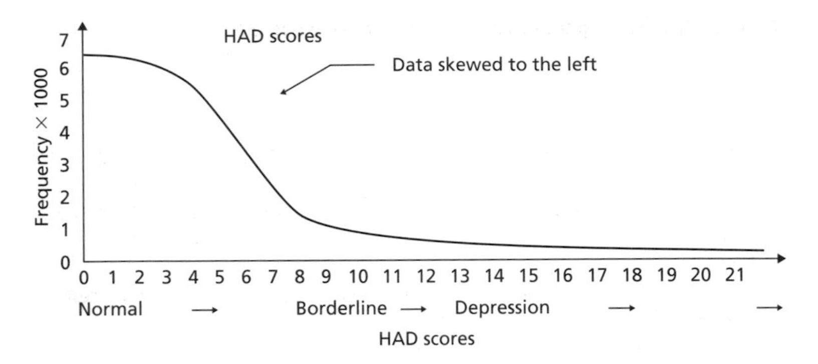

Figure 1.11 Depression scores on the 'Hospital Anxiety and Depression' (HAD) scale obtained from 100 randomly selected people from the general population shows skewed data.

either be transformed into a Normal-ish distribution by taking powers, reciprocals or logarithms of data values or, alternatively, researchers may apply statistical tests that need not work with an assumption of normality and these are called 'non-parametric' statistical tests (Figure 1.11). The danger with the approach of transforming data is that the results of any analysis will no longer refer to the original data values (e.g. mean values) and will therefore be difficult to interpret.

As statistical tools, non-parametric tests are generally not as powerful as their parametric counterparts. This weakness arises from the fact that they are usually associated with larger *p*-values compared to the parametric tests, in particular when applied to small-sized samples. In other words, with non-parametric tests there is a higher likelihood of making a Type II error.

Although deemed less flexible and less powerful than parametric tests, non-parametric tests are never the less indispensable statistical tools to be used with skewed data. The non-parametric tests used when comparing mean or median values from two groups are the 'Mann–Whitney U test' (*unpaired data*) and the 'Wilcoxon signed-rank test' (*paired data*).

Unpaired versus paired data

When data to be compared have been gathered from independent samples without any indication that data were paired in any way, unpaired statistical tests should be used in the analysis. Unpaired tests are the χ^2 test

Table 1.5 Summarizing the different uses of the statistical tests

Testing for difference	Normal continuous data	Skewed continuous data/ discrete numerical data/ ranked categorical data	Binary categorical data
With one sample	One-sample *t*-test	Wilcoxon signed rank test	χ^2 test (or Fisher's exact test)
Between two independent samples	*t*-test	Mann–Whitney U test	χ^2 test (or Fisher's exact test)
Between two paired samples	Paired *t*-test	Wilcoxon matched pairs test	McNemar's test
Between three or more independent samples	ANOVA	Kruskal–Wallis test	χ^2 test
Between three or more paired samples	ANOVA	Friedman test	McNemar's test

(*categorical data*), unpaired *t*-test (*continuous Normally distributed data*) and the Mann–Whitney U test (*continuous non-Normally distributed data*).

When data to be compared have been gathered in such a way as to be seen to occur in pairs, the paired statistical tests should be used. These instances would include respective before-and-after or left-side–right-side measurements in a set of individuals, twin studies and certain matched case-control studies.

Paired tests are the McNemar's test (*binary data*) paired *t*-test (*continuous Normally distributed data*) and the Wilcoxon signed-rank test (*continuous non-Normally distributed data*).

Tests used with single or several samples

The continuous-data tests discussed so far are all used (as indicated) in the comparison of data obtained from two groups in order to test for a significant difference.

Data obtained from only one sample can be analysed by use of the one-sample *t*-test (*Normal data*) or the Wilcoxon test (*non-Normal data*). In these one-sample tests, mean or median values obtained from a single sample are compared with theoretical mean or median values, respectively.

In studies where three or more groups are being compared, the ANOVA test (*Normal data*) or the Kruskal–Wallis test (*non-Normal data*) are the appropriate statistical instruments to use (see Table 1.5).

Correlation and regression

The following sections on correlation and regression methods have been prepared specifically for the purposes of critical appraisal and are by no means a complete treatment of this complicated subject area. Interested readers may wish to consult the more formal statistical texts.

Correlation

Correlation describes a simple statistical procedure that examines whether a linear association exists between two different independent variables, X and Y. Correlation is used when both compared variables have simply been measured and their values have not been controlled or pre-set in any way.

For example, if variables such as blood pressure and serum cholesterol were measured in a randomly selected sample of, say, 50 individuals from the general population, correlation can be used to test for a possible linear association that may exist between them.

The magnitude and direction of any identified linear associations are expressed as a correlation co-efficient. A positive correlation means that Y increases linearly with X, and a negative correlation means that Y decreases linearly as X increases. Zero correlation reflects a complete non-association between the compared variables.

The correlation co-efficient is usually presented with appropriate *p*-values and confidence intervals.

Pearson's correlation co-efficient (*r*)

When the two variables being examined are numerical and continuous in nature, the Pearson's correlation co-efficient '*r*' is the appropriate measure of correlation to use. The Pearson's correlation co-efficient *r* can take any value within a range of -1 to $+1$.

The Pearson's correlation co-efficient can only be used to test for linear associations between two continuous variables whose data follow a Normal distribution. If these conditions are not fulfilled by the data, other measures of correlation should be used instead. Also, correlation should only really be employed in cases where it is unclear as to which is the independent variable (X) and which is the dependent variable (Y).

Correlation, not causation!

The concept of an association between two variables must be distinguished from that of causation, which plays no part when discussing correlation. In other words, with correlation we are not interested in a causal relationship between blood pressure and serum cholesterol; we are simply interested in quantifying how well they vary together. If we were interested in causality, we would need to employ a different statistical test, such as regression.

Note that even when X and Y are seen as showing a strong correlation, explanations can include any of the following:

- X partly determines the value of Y.
- Y partly determines the value of X.
- A third confounding variable is responsible for corresponding changes in X and Y.
- A mere chance observation.

Consider the following possible correlations between continuous variables X and Y (Figure 1.12).

Formula for the Pearson's correlation co-efficient

$$r = \frac{\Sigma(x - \overline{x})(y - \overline{y})}{\sqrt{\Sigma(x - \overline{x})^2 (y - \overline{y})^2}}$$

r is usually presented with an accompanying p-value which address the following question: If no correlation exists between the two variables under consideration, that is, $r = 0$, what is the probability of obtaining by pure chance, a value of r as far away from zero as observed with these data?

r Square

Variability is bound to be present in any data set, for example the blood pressure values obtained from our 50 volunteers. This inevitable variability in blood pressure values would probably have been due to a host of factors, such as genetic differences, dietary differences, racial differences, body weight differences, serum cholesterol differences and even mere chance random variation.

Therefore, when testing two different variables for a possible correlation, r^2 can be thought of as being the part of the variability observed in

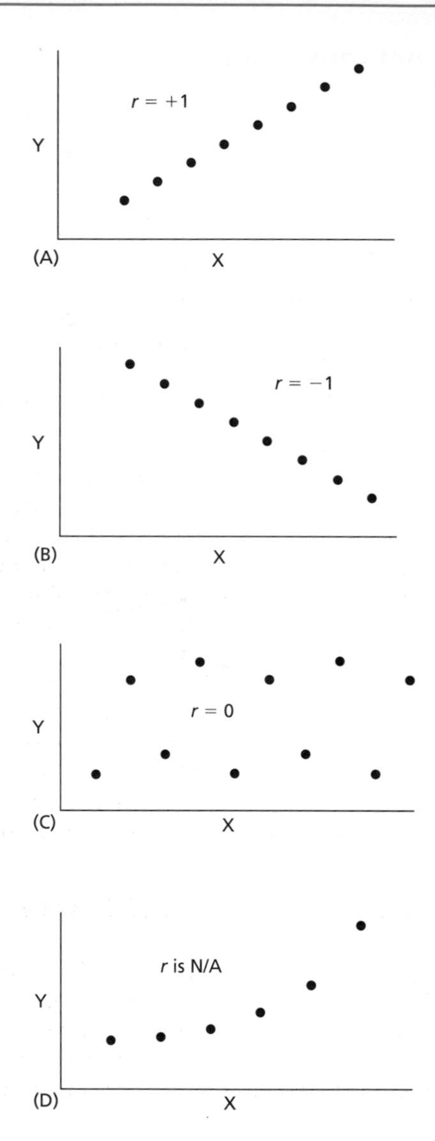

Figure 1.12 Scatter plots of different correlations. (A) $r = +1$ denotes a perfect positive linear relationship where an increase in X is accompanied by an equal increase in Y; (B) $r = -1$ denotes a perfect inverse linear relationship where an increase in X is accompanied by an equal decrease in Y; (C) $r = 0$ denotes a complete lack of correlation between the two continuous variables being considered; (D) The Pearson's correlation coefficient r is not applicable with such curved plots, that is, non-linear relationships. In such instances, other measures are used instead.

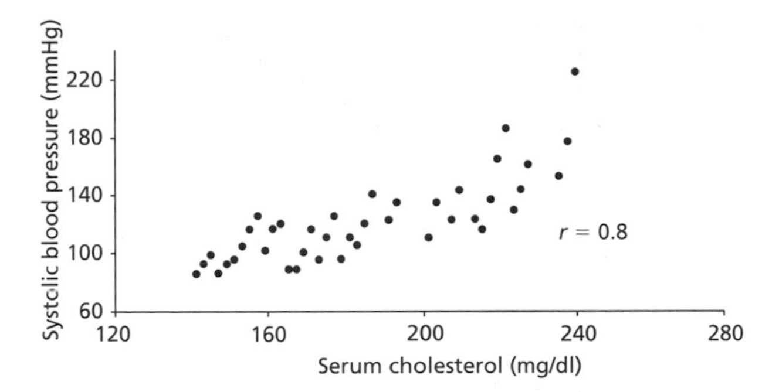

Figure 1.13 Correlation between blood pressure and serum cholesterol in 50 volunteers.

the values of one variable that can be directly ascribed to the effects of the other variable. With most data, value of r^2 lies between 0 and 1.

With our example, r^2 would represent the fraction of the variability observed with blood pressure values that was actually due to serum cholesterol differences, or the fraction of the variability observed with serum cholesterol values that was actually due to blood pressure differences amongst the 50 volunteers (Figure 1.13).

From the data obtained from our 50 volunteers, $r = 0.8$ and therefore $r^2 = 0.64$. This means that only 64% of the variability observed with blood pressure values can be explained by serum cholesterol differences and vice versa. The remaining 36% of the variability would probably have been due to other factors such as those described above.

Note: r^2 is only used with the Pearson's correlation co-efficient.

Spearman's rank correlation co-efficient (ρ)

When examining continuous data that do not follow a Normal distribution, or when data being considered are discrete or ordinal in nature, another correlation co-efficient called the 'Spearman's rank correlation co-efficient ρ' is used instead. As suggested by its name, the 'Spearman's ρ' is calculated by use of the ranks of data observations.

Formula for the Spearman's rank correlation co-efficient

$$\rho = 1 - \frac{6\Sigma d^2}{n^3 - n}$$

Table 1.6 Ranked weight and serum cholesterol data from 10 volunteers

Subject	Cholesterol rank	Blood pressure rank	Difference in ranks (*d*)	d^2
1	1	3	−2	4
2	2	9	−7	49
3	3	8	−5	25
4	4	2	2	4
5	5	6	−1	1
6	6	1	5	25
7	7	10	−3	9
8	8	7	1	1
9	9	4	5	25
10	10	5	5	25

ρ is also presented with an accompanying *p*-value which addresses the following question: If the null hypothesis were true and no correlation exists between the two variables under consideration, that is, $\rho = 0$, what is the probability of obtaining by pure chance, a value of ρ as far away from zero as observed in this experiment?

Attempt to calculate the Spearman's ρ using the cholesterol and body weight data gathered from these 10 subjects using the formula provided. According to the data (Table 1.6), Spearman's rank correlation co-efficient $\rho = -0.02$.

Linear regression

The example used throughout this section examines the relationship between body weight (X) and serum cholesterol (Y) based on data gathered from our 50 randomly picked volunteers.

Rather than just measuring the strength of correlation between two independent data sets, linear regression is used to examine the exact nature of the linear relationship that may exist between X and Y. Usually, regression is used when it is fairly clear between the compared variables, which is the independent variable X, and which is the dependent variable Y. The values of X may have even been controlled or pre-set in the experiment.

As shown in Figure 1.14, linear regression works by finding the straight line that best explains the relationship between the X and Y data sets, so that for a given value of X, a corresponding value of Y can be predicted. This is called 'data modelling'.

Casual attempts to draw lines through a scatter plot would inevitably result in many data observations falling above and below those lines.

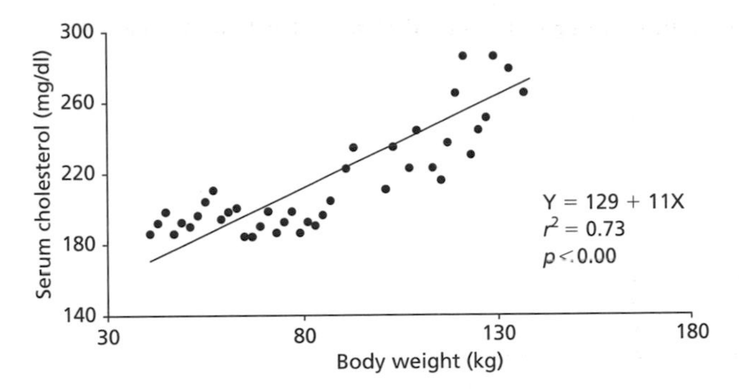

Figure 1.14 Scatter plot of two variables X (body weight) and Y (serum cholesterol).

However, the linear regression line can be described as that which results in the least combined distance between the data points and the line. In other words, a 'best-fit' linear regression line.

REGRESSION LINE BY LEAST-SQUARES METHOD

The linear regression procedure starts out by drawing several tentative lines through the scatter plot. At each attempt, the vertical distance (S) of each data observation from the tentative line is measured and squared (S^2). All squared distances are then added together to produce a 'sum-of-squared-distances' measure (S^2) for that tentative line. The eventual linear regression line is determined by finding the line that results in the least 'sum-of-squared-distances' (S^2).

The linear regression equation

As described above, a linear regression line is used to model the relationship between variables X and Y. This linear model tells us how Y changes with X, thereby making it possible to predict the value of Y for any given value of X. This linear model can be represented algebraically as a linear regression equation (Figure 1.15).

According to the serum cholesterol and body weight model in Figure 1.14, $Y = 129 + 11X$. The given value of 11 for the 'regression co-efficient *b*' means that, according to these data, serum cholesterol increases by 11 mg/dl for every 1 kg increase in body weight.

The regression co-efficient *b* is usually presented along with 95% confidence intervals and a *p*-value, which addresses the question: If the null

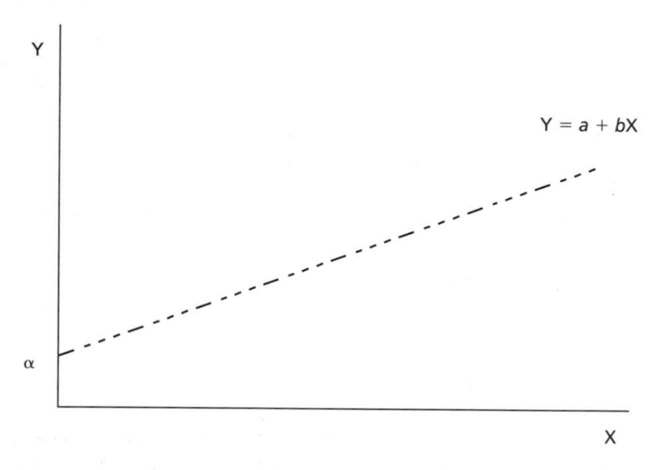

Figure 1.15 The linear regression equation. Y = dependent (response) variable; X = independent (predictor) variable; *a* = intercept (i.e. value of Y when X is zero); *b* = gradient of recession line (i.e. the change in Y for a unit change in X).

hypothesis were true and $b = 0$ (i.e. Y is absolutely not determined by X), what is the probability of obtaining by pure chance, a value of b as far away from zero as observed with these data?

Note: the linear regression model is only applicable over the range of X variable measurements made. In other words, the regression line should never be extrapolated in any direction because linearity of the relationship cannot be assumed in these uncharted territories. Moreover, by extrapolating the regression line, data values may be rendered meaningless. Have you ever met anyone with a body weight of 1 kg or a serum cholesterol value of −40 mg/dl?

Goodness-of-fit

Interestingly, the square of the Pearson's correlation co-efficient r^2 is usually also computed from the data in a regression analysis to express how well the linear model fits in with the observed data. Here, r^2 can be thought of as being the part of the total variation in Y that can be explained by the regression model. With most data, the value of r^2 lies between 0 and 1.

According to our data, $r^2 = 0.73$. This means that our linear regression model accounted for 73% of the variation observed with the serum cholesterol data (Figure 1.16).

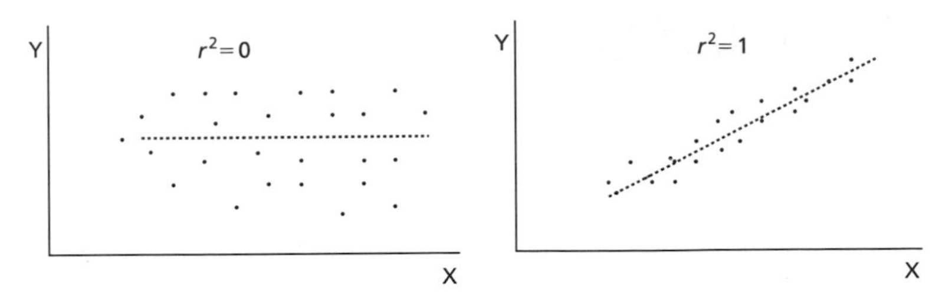

Figure 1.16 Goodness-of-fit by r^2.

Multiple linear regression

With simple linear regression, the relationship between the dependent variable Y and the independent variable X is explained by use of a linear model $Y = a + bX$. In the real world, however, the value of the dependent variable Y may well be influenced by many independent variables operating simultaneously.

Thankfully, the linear model can be extended to incorporate several independent variables to show how they all influence the value of Y. A multiple regression model can be summarized as $Y = a + b_1X_1 + b_2X_2 + b_3X_3 + \cdots + b_kX_k$.

INTERPRETATION OF THE MULTIPLE REGRESSION MODEL

- a = value of Y when all independent variables are zero.
- b_1, b_2 and b_3, called 'partial regression co-efficients' are similarly determined by the least-squares method.
- For each unit increase in X_1, Y increases by an amount equivalent to b_1 provided $X_2, X_3, \ldots, X_k$ remain constant.
- For each unit increase in X_2, Y increases by an amount equivalent to b_2 provided $X_1, X_3, \ldots, X_k$ remain constant.
- For each unit increase in X_3, Y increases by an amount equivalent to b_3 provided $X_1, X_3, \ldots, X_k$ remain constant.

Multiple regression is a frequently used technique that allows researchers to explore the effects that a number of variables may have on the outcome of a study, and also to control for possible confounding factors that may be present in a study. Multiple regression can also be a useful tool to have when developing a prognostic index for a particular disorder.

Extending our serum cholesterol and body weight example, we may want to consider the possible effect of 'age' and 'exercise' on the serum

Table 1.7 Entering all data into a statistical package would produce multiple regression results such as below

Variable		Regression coefficient (a, b)	95% CI (a, b)	*p*-value
Constant	a	12	−1.6 to 24.8	0.8
Body weight	b_1	8.4	6.1 to 10.7	0.000
Age	b_2	29.4	9.9 to 48.9	0.006
Exercise	b_3	−14.9	−6.2 to −23.6	0.001

Dependent variable: serum cholesterol.

cholesterol data. Being continuous in nature, age data can be incorporated into the multiple regression analysis in a straightforward way.

However, imagine that the exercise data were gathered in a categorical 'active or sedentary' format. In order to incorporate such categorical data into our multiple regression model, the 'active' and 'sedentary' categories would have to be assigned *dummy* variables, for example sedentary = 0 and active = 1 (Table 1.7).

Multiple regression equation

$$Y = 12 + (8.4 \times \text{body weight}) + (29.4 \times \text{age}) + (-14.9 \times \text{exercise status})$$

Interpretation:

- For every 1 kg increase in body weight, serum cholesterol increases by 8.4 mg/dl for the same age and exercise status ($p < 0.01$), that is, significant relationship between body weight and serum cholesterol.
- For every one-year increase in age, serum cholesterol increases by 29.4 mg/dl for the same body weight and exercise status ($p < 0.01$), that is, significant relationship between age and serum cholesterol.
- Given the same body weight and age, those who are physically active have a serum cholesterol level 14.9 mg/dl lower than those who lead a sedentary lifestyle ($p < 0.01$), that is, significant inverse relationship between exercise and serum cholesterol.

Some readers may find it helpful to read about 'odds' and 'odds ratios' in Chapter 6 before continuing with the next section.

Logistic regression

Logistic regression is used in data sets where the dependent variable Y is binary in nature, such as *dead/alive, stroke/no-stroke* categories. This is in contrast to linear regression, which is used when Y is a continuous variable.

When considering binary outcomes, such as *event/non-event* outcomes, in logistic regression, our clinical interest actually lies in determining the risk (π) of developing an event, given a set of values for the independent variable(s) X. We may also want to know how these independent variables influence the risk (π) of that event.

Therefore the logistic regression model can be described as that which examines the relationship between one or more independent variables $X_1, X_2, X_3, \ldots, X_k$ and the risk (π) of developing an event Y.

However, there are mathematical problems with working with risk values as a dependent variable Y. This is because in contrast to the continuous dependent variable Y seen with linear regression, risk values are restricted to values of between 0 and 1 and mathematically, this is an unworkable constraint.

Thankfully, risk values can be transformed in such a way as to be completely unrestricted, taking any value between $-\infty$ to $+\infty$, just like with any continuous variable. This is done by what is called a 'logit transformation of risk'.

LOGIT TRANSFORMATION OF RISK

- Convert risk (π) of events to odds of event = $\pi/1 - \pi$.
- Convert odds of event ($\pi/1 - \pi$) to $\text{Log}_e(\pi/1 - \pi)$.
- Log_e odds of event can range from $-\infty$ to $+\infty$ just like a continuous numerical variable.

Therefore, in logistic regression, Y = Log_e odds of event.

To summarize, we have said that logistic regression is used when Y is a binary outcome, for example *event/non-event*. We have also said that with binary outcomes, the focus of interest is actually in knowing the risk (π) of developing an event. However, a risk measure is limited to a range of 0–1.

Therefore, a logit transformation of risk is performed in order to create the Log_e odds of an event. This transforms a binary outcome variable to a measure that can operate mathematically like a continuous variable, being able to take any value between $-\infty$ and $+\infty$. This is the essence of logistic regression.

Logistic regression formula and interpretation

For one independent variable:

$$\text{Log}_e \text{ odds of event Y} = a + bX$$

Table 1.8 Entering all data into a statistical package provides multiple regression results as below

Variable		Regression coefficient (a, b)	95% CI (a, b)	$\exp^{(b)}$	*p*-value
Constant	a	−1.342	–	0.25	0.23
Serum cholesterol	b_1	0.17	0.10 to 0.24	1.2	0.03
Body weight	b_2	0.23	0.12 to 0.34	1.3	0.01
Age	b_3	0.08	−0.41 to 0.57	1.1	0.4
Exercise	b_4	−1.76	−1.83 to −1.69	0.02	0.00

Dependent variable: Log_e odds myocardial infarction (MI).

For K independent variables:

$$\text{Log}_e \text{ odds of event Y} = a + b_1X_1 + b_2X_2 + b_3X_3 + \cdots + b_kX_k$$

Because of the logit transformation that is applied to original risk values in logistic regression, the co-efficients $b_1, b_2, b_3, \ldots, b_k$ are actually related to the Log_e odds of event Y (see above formulae). Therefore, in order to find how the respective independent variables $X_1, \ldots, X_k$ directly affect the actual odds of event Y, the antilog of these co-efficients, that is, $\exp^{(b_1)}, \exp^{(b_2)}, \exp^{(b_3)}, \ldots, \exp^{(b_k)}$, would need to be determined.

In other words, in logistic regression, $\exp^{(b)}$ and not '*b*' represents the 'increase in odds' of event Y associated with a unit increase in X.

To complicate life further, some logistic regression models can also feature a binary independent variable X. Under such circumstances, the binary variable is assigned dummy variables in order to be incorporated into the logistic regression model.

However, the $\exp^{(b)}$ value derived with such a binary X variable would actually represent the odds ratio of event Y when $X = 1$ (i.e. not an 'increase in odds' of event Y as is the case with continuous X variables).

Example: The example used here (Table 1.8) examines the relationship between the risk of a myocardial infarction (*binary outcome Y*) and the independent variables of body weight (X_1), serum cholesterol (X_2), age (X_3) and exercise (X_4) based on data gathered from our 50 volunteers.

Logistic regression equation

$$\text{Log}_e \text{ odds of event Y} = -3.42 + (0.17 \times \text{serum cholesterol}) + (0.23 \times \text{body weight}) + (0.08 \times \text{age}) + (-1.76 \times \text{exercise status})$$

Interpretation:

- For every 1 mg/dl increase in serum cholesterol, odds of myocardial infarction (MI) event increase by 1.2($\exp^{0.17}$) for the same weight, age, and exercise status ($p = 0.03$), that is, signficant relationship between serum cholesterol and odds of MI.
- For every 1 kg increase in body weight, odds of MI event increase by 1.3($\exp^{0.23}$) for the same cholesterol level, age and exercise status ($p = 0.01$), that is, significant relationship between body weight and odds of MI.
- For every one-year increase in age, odds of MI event increase by 1.1($\exp^{0.08}$) for the same cholesterol level, body weight and exercise status ($p < 0.40$), that is, non-significant relationship between age and odds of MI.
- Given the same cholesterol level, body weight and age, the odds ratio of MI event is 0.2($\exp^{-1.76}$) for those who exercise compared to those who are sedentary ($p < 0.01$), that is, significant inverse relationship between exercise and odds of MI. Here, $\exp^{(b)}$ is an odds ratio because exercise status is a binary variable.

Non-essential information

The chi-square test

CONDITIONS

Any number of groups; categorical data.

ESSENCE

Categorical data from different samples are compared regarding any real differences. (Note: categorical data from a single sample can be compared with a theoretical ideal.)

NULL HYPOTHESIS

No real differences exist between categorical data obtained from different samples and, as such, these samples belong to the same population.

ALTERNATIVE HYPOTHESIS

Categorical data obtained from compared samples are too different for these samples to belong to the same population.

The example used here is that of a retrospective study in which 98 lung cancer patients and 102 control subjects were assessed for a past history of smoking.

	Observed data (O)			Expected data (E)		
	Lung cancer patients	Control subjects	Total	Lung cancer patients	Control subjects	Total
Smoker	72	44	116	57	59	116
Non-smoker	26	58	84	41	43	84
Total	98	102	200	98	102	200

THE CHI-SQUARE TEST

- Calculate the expected numbers for each cell. This can be calculated for each cell according to the formula (Row total) × (Column total)/ table total, for example expected number for cell 'a'
$$= (116 \times 98)/200 = 57.$$
- For each cell, calculate: $(O - E)^2/E$, for example for cell 'a',
$$(O - E)^2/E = (72 - 57)^2/E = 18.482.$$
- The chi-square statistic is obtained by adding values of all $(O-E)^2/E$ obtained from every cell: $X^2 = (O - E)^2/E$. According to our data,
$$X^2 = (O - E)^2/E = 18.482.$$
- The degrees of freedom (*df*) in a categorical data set can be determined by the formula: df = (Number of rows − 1) × (Number of columns − 1). According to our data, $df = 1$.

Looking along the $df = 1$ row in Table, $\chi^2 = 18.482$ is greater than the figure quoted for a probability of 0.001. Therefore, $p < 0.001$.

P-value expresses the probability of obtaining categorical data as discrepant as observed, if no difference existed between the compared samples. The probability of such discrepant data in light of a true null hypothesis is one in 1000. The null hypothesis has been disproved.

The one-sample test

CONDITIONS

One-sample data; Normal data.

ESSENCE

Sample mean ($\bar{x}$) is compared with a theoretical or hypothetical population mean (μ).

NULL HYPOTHESIS

Sample from which mean ($\bar{x}$) was derived belongs to the same population from which population mean (μ) was derived.

ALTERNATIVE HYPOTHESIS

Sample mean ($\bar{x}$) is too different from population mean (μ) that the sample cannot be said to belong to the same population from which population mean (μ) was derived.

Assuming $\mu = 2$, consider the postman data set where $\bar{x} = 5.25$ with a standard deviation of 10.77.

Sorted responses from the survey of postmen																			
0	0	0	1	1	1	1	2	2	**2**	**3**	4	4	4	4	5	6	6	6	7	50

ONE-SAMPLE *t*-TEST

- Population mean (μ) = 2.
- Sample mean ($\bar{x}$) = 5.25.
- Difference between means ($-\bar{x}$) = -3.25. (Note: Negative sign is disregarded.)
- Sample standard deviation (SD) = 10.77
- Number of observations (n) = 20.
- Degrees of freedom (df) = ($n - 1$) = 19. (Used in t-tests to allow for the effects of sample size on standard error.)
- Standard error of sample mean (SE) = $\text{SD}/n = 2/4$.

The t statistic is similar to the z statistic used earlier for very large samples; t = how many standard errors is the difference between means?

$$t = (-\bar{x})/\text{SE} = 3.25/2.4 = 1.354$$

Looking along the $df = 19$ row in Table i, $t = 1.354$ falls between a probability of 0.5 and 0.1 ($0.1 < p < 0.5$). Therefore, $p < 0.5$.

P-value expresses the probability of obtaining a mean value as far away from the population mean as observed. If a random sample was taken from the population from which population mean (μ) was derived.

The Wilcoxon rank sum test

CONDITIONS

One-sample data; skewed data.

ESSENCE

Sample median (m) is compared with a theoretical or hypothetical mean (μ).

NULL HYPOTHESIS

Sample from which median (m) was derived belongs to the same population from which hypothetical mean (μ) was derived.

ALTERNATIVE HYPOTHESIS

Sample median (m) is too different from hypothetical mean (μ) that the sample cannot be said to belong to the same population from which hypothetical mean (μ) was derived.

Assuming $\mu = 2$, consider the postman data set where $m = 2.5$.

Sorted responses from the survey of postmen regarding the number of dog attacks																			
0	0	0	1	1	1	1	2	2	**2**	**3**	4	4	4	5	6	6	6	7	50

THE WILCOXON RANK SUM TEST

- All observations where $x = \mu$ are discarded.
- For all remaining data observations, respective distances from the median are calculated ($m - x$).
- All distances ($m - x$) are ranked from low to high.
- The lowest rank = 1 and the highest rank = n (number of remaining observations).
- ($m - x$) having the same value are assigned a mean of their ranks.
- With observations where $x < \mu$ ranks are assigned a negative sign ($\gamma-$).
- With observations where $x > \mu$ ranks are assigned a postive sign (γ).
- Sum all negative ranks ($\Sigma\gamma-$).
- Sum all positive ranks ($\Sigma\gamma$).
- Add both sums together ($\Sigma\gamma-$) + ($\Sigma\gamma$), should equal 97 with the postman data set.

If null hypothesis is correct then $(\Sigma\gamma-) + (\Sigma\gamma) = 0$ (or near zero). The farther away from zero $(\Sigma\gamma-) + (\Sigma\gamma)$ is, the smaller the *p*-value. *P*-value expresses the probability of obtaining a $(\Sigma\gamma-) + (\Sigma\ \gamma)$ value as far away from zero as observed, if a random sample was taken from the population from which hypothetical mean (μ) was derived.

The *t*-test

CONDITIONS

Two independent samples; Normal data; unpaired data.

ESSENCE

'Sample a' mean ($\bar{x}$a) is compared with 'Sample b' mean ($\bar{x}$b).

NULL HYPOTHESIS

Sample a mean ($\bar{x}$a) is not that different from Sample b mean ($\bar{x}$b) and both samples belong to the same population (i.e. a = b).

ALTERNATIVE HYPOTHESIS

Sample a mean ($\bar{x}$a) is too different from Sample b mean ($\bar{x}$b) for both samples to belong to the same population (i.e. a ≠ b).

Using the height data:

Sample a	Sample b
Mean height ($\bar{x}$a) = 170 cm	Mean height ($\bar{x}$b) = 160 cm
Standard deviation (SDa) = 9.5 cm	Standard deviation (SDb) = 13 cm
Number in sample (*n*a) = 100	Number in sample (*n*b) = 100
Degrees of freedom (*df*) = (*n*a − 1) = 99	Degrees of freedom (*df*) = (*n*b − 1) = 99

INDEPENDENT SAMPLES *t*-TEST

Difference between sample means ($\bar{x}$a − $\bar{x}$b) = 10 cm. Let us assume that a statistic which we shall call 'K':

$$\frac{(n\text{a} - 1)\text{SDa} + (n\text{b} - 1)\text{SDb}}{(n\text{a} + n\text{b}) - 2}$$

Then, the standard error (SE) of ($\bar{x}$a − $\bar{x}$b) can be calculated according to the formula:

$$\sqrt{\frac{K}{n\mathrm{a}} + \frac{K}{n\mathrm{b}}} = \sqrt{\frac{11}{99} + \frac{11}{99}} = 0.48$$

The t statistic is similar to the z statistic used earlier for very large samples. Therefore, the t statistic, that is, how many standard errors is the mean difference = 10 cm/0.48 = 20.8. Looking along the $df = 66$ row in Table $t = 20.8$ falls below a probability of 0.001. Therefore, $p < 0.001$.

P-value expresses the probability of obtaining a difference in mean values as large as observed if both samples were taken from the same population.

CONCLUSION

If both sets of men were really from the same population and no real difference existed between them regarding mean height, the probability of obtaining results as discrepant as these is less than one in 1000 ($p < 1000$) and therefore, the null hypothesis is rejected.

In other words, the height difference between both samples is too large for us to believe that both samples came from the same population.

The Mann–Whitney U test

CONDITIONS

Two independent samples; skewed/discrete data; unpaired data.

ESSENCE

Sample a median (*m*a) is compared with Sample b median (*m*b).

NULL HYPOTHESIS

Sample a median (*m*a) is not that different from Sample b median (*m*b) and both samples belong to the same population (i.e. a = b).

ALTERNATIVE HYPOTHESIS

Sample a median (*m*a) is too different from Sample b median (*m*b) for both samples to belong to the same population (i.e. a ≠ b).

Consider that the following postmen data sets were obtained from two different districts 'a' and 'b'.

Sorted responses from the survey of postmen regarding number of dog attacks – District a																			
0	0	0	1	1	1	1	2	2	**2**	**3**	4	4	4	5	6	6	6	7	50

Sorted responses from the survey of postmen regarding number of dog attacks – District b																			
0	0	0	0	1	1	1	1	1	**1**	**1**	1	1	1	2	2	5	5	6	6

THE MANN–WHITNEY U TEST

- Mix *all* data observations from both groups together.
- Rank *all* observations from low to high regardless of group.
- Data observation with smallest value is assigned the lowest rank = 1.
- Data observation with biggest value is assigned the highest rank = n (i.e. the combined number of observations in both groups).
- Observations (x) having the same value are assigned a mean of their ranks.
- Having assigned a rank to each data observation, sum all group 'a' ranks ($\Sigma\gamma a$).
- Sum all group 'b' ranks ($\Sigma\gamma b$).
- Summed ranks ($\Sigma\gamma a$) and ($\Sigma\gamma b$) = 0 (or near zero).
- If null hypothesis is correct then $(\Sigma\gamma a) - (\Sigma\gamma b) = 0$ (or near zero).

The larger the value of $(\Sigma\gamma a) - (\Sigma\gamma b)$, the smaller the p-value, which can be read off appropriate statistical tables. P-value expresses the probability of obtaining sum of rank values as discrepant as observed if both samples were taken from the same population.

The paired *t*-test

CONDITIONS

Two samples; Normal data; paired data.

ESSENCE

Sample a mean ($\bar{x}$a) is compared with Sample b mean ($\bar{x}$b) with both samples being paired.

The example used here is that of a clinical trial in which 10 bilateral diabetic simple leg ulcer patients received two different kinds of dressing, that is, one for each ulcer for the duration of a month, after which the extent of wound healed (cm) was measured for both ulcers in every patient.

NULL HYPOTHESIS

Treatment a mean ($\bar{x}$a) is not different from Treatment b mean ($\bar{x}$b) and both treatments are equivalent, i.e. (a = b).

ALTERNATIVE HYPOTHESIS

Treatment a mean ($\bar{x}$a) is too different from Treatment b mean ($\bar{x}$b) for both treatments to be equivalent, i.e. (a $\neq$ b).

Subject	1	2	3	4	5	6	7	8	9	10
Treatment a	10	7	2	8	4	8	4	6	3	9
Treatment b	7	2	3	8	2	8	7	3	8	8
Pair difference (*d*)	3	5	−1	0	2	0	−3	3	−5	1

THE PAIRED *t*-TEST

- Mean of pair differences ($\bar{d}$) = 0.5.
- Degrees of freedom (*df*) ($n - 1$) = 9.
- Standard deviation (SD) of pair differences:

$$\sqrt{\frac{(\Sigma\bar{d} - d)^2}{n - 1}} = 7.7$$

- Standard error (SE) of pair differences:

$$\frac{\text{SD}}{\sqrt{n}} = 2.44$$

- Therefore, the *t* statistic, that is, how many standard errors is the mean of pair differences $t = \bar{d}/\text{SE} = 0.0002$.

Looking along the $df = 9$ row in Table, $t = 0.002$ falls below a probability of 0.5. Therefore, $p < 0.5$ (or less than one in two).

P-value expresses a probability of obtaining a difference in mean values as large as observed if both samples were taken from the same population.

CONCLUSION

If both sets of treatments were really equivalent, the probability of obtaining results as discrepant as these is less than one in two ($p < 0.5$) and, therefore, the null hypothesis cannot be discarded!

In other words, the pair differences obtained with both treatments are not sufficiently different for us to conclude that both treatments are not equivalent.

The Wilcoxon matched-pairs signed rank test

CONDITIONS

Two samples; skewed/discrete data; paired data.

ESSENCE

Sample a median (ma) is compared with Sample b median (mb).

NULL HYPOTHESIS

Treatment a median (ma) is no different from Treatment b median (mb) and both treatments are equivalent, i.e. (a = b).

ALTERNATIVE HYPOTHESIS

Treatment a mean (xa) is too different from Treatment b mean (xb) for both treatments to be equivalent, i.e. (a ≠ b).

The example used here is that of a clinical trial in which 10 bilateral diabetic simple leg ulcer patients received two different kinds of dressing, that is, one for each ulcer for the duration of a month, after which the extent of wound healed (cm) was measured for both ulcers in every patient.

Subject	1	2	3	4	5	6	7	8	9	10
Treatment a	10	7	2	8	4	8	4	6	3	9
Treatment b	7	2	3	8	2	8	7	3	8	8
Pair difference (d)	3	5	−1	0	2	0	−3	3	−5	1

THE WILCOXON MATCHED-PAIRS SIGNED RANK TEST

- Calculate pair differences for all subjects.
- Ignoring any minus signs present, rank *all* pair differences from low to high.
- Data observation with smallest value is assigned the lowest rank = 1.

- Data observation with biggest value is assigned the highest rank = n (i.e. the total number of paired observations).
- Observations (x) having the same value are assigned a mean of their ranks.
- Having assigned a rank to each data observation, sum all ranks for which Treatment a was superior ($\Sigma\gamma$a).
- Sum all ranks for which Treatment b was superior ($\Sigma\gamma$b).
- Summed ranks ($\Sigma\gamma$a) and ($\Sigma\gamma$b) = 0 (or near zero).

If null hypothesis is correct then ($\Sigma\gamma$a) − ($\Sigma\gamma$b) = 0 (or near zero). The larger the value of ($\Sigma\gamma$a) − ($\Sigma\gamma$b), the smaller the p-value, which can be read off appropriate statistical tables. P-value expresses the probability of obtaining sum of rank values as discrepant as observed if both treatments were really equivalent.

The analysis of variance (ANOVA) test

CONDITIONS

Three or more samples; Normal data; unpaired data.

ESSENCE

Sample means are compared from groups a, b, c, …, z.

NULL HYPOTHESIS

No difference exists between the compared groups, which all belong to the same population.

ALTERNATIVE HYPOTHESIS

A difference exists between the compared groups and the groups do not come from the same population.

The example used here is that of a clinical trial in which 20 depressed patients were randomized to receive one of the treatments listed below. Improvements, as reflected by HAD questionnaire scores, were assessed after three months.

	(a) Tricyclic (n = 5)	(b) SSRI (n = 5)	(c) CBT (n = 5)	(d) IPT (n = 5)
Improvements in scores (x)	3	16	13	12
	6	12	10	8
	7	13	10	8
	7	9	5	13
	10	12	7	6
Mean improvement ($\bar{x}$)	6.6	12.4	9	5.3

Overall mean ($\overline{x}_t$):

$$= \frac{\overline{x}_a + \overline{x}_b + \overline{x}_c + \cdots + \overline{x}_z}{N}$$

N = number of groups;
n = number of observations within a group.

THE ANOVA TEST

- Compares variability between group means with variability of observations within the groups.
- Variability within each group (V)

$$= \frac{\Sigma(\overline{x} - x)^2}{n - 1}$$

(Note: Variance has been used here instead of standard deviation.)
- Combined within-group variability (C^V)

$$= \frac{V_a(n_a - 1) + V_b(n_b - 1) + V_c(n_c - 1) + \cdots + V_z(n_z - 1)}{nN - N}$$

- Between group variability (B^V)

$$= \frac{n_a(\overline{x}_t - \overline{x}_a)^2 + n_b(\overline{x}_t - \overline{x}_b)^2 + n_c(\overline{x}_t - \overline{x}_c)^2 + \cdots + n_z(\overline{x}_t - \overline{x}_z)^2}{nN - 1}$$

- F statistic

$$= \frac{B^V}{C^V}$$

If the null hypothesis was correct, $F = 1$ (or close to 1). The larger the value of F, the smaller the p-value. The p-value expresses the probability of obtaining such discrepant mean values in the compared groups if all compared groups really belonged to the same population.

The Kruskal–Wallis test

CONDITIONS

Three or more samples; skewed/discrete data; unpaired data.

ESSENCE

Sample medians are compared from groups a, b, c, …, z.

NULL HYPOTHESIS

No difference exists between the sample medians obtained from all compared groups and all groups belong to the same population.

ALTERNATIVE HYPOTHESIS

A difference exists between the sample medians observed in all compared groups and these respective samples are too different to have come from the same population.

The example used here is that of a clinical trial in which 20 depressed patients were randomized to receive one of the treatments listed below. Improvements, as reflected by HAD questionnaire scores, were assessed after three months.

	Placebo (n = 5)	SSRI (n = 5)	CBT (n = 5)	IPT (n = 5)
HAD questionnaire improvement scores after 3 months	3	16	13	12
	6	12	10	8
	7	13	10	14
	7	9	5	13
	10	12	7	6

THE KRUSKAL–WALLIS TEST

- Mix data observations from *all* groups together.
- Rank *all* observations from low to high regardless of group.
- Data observation with smallest value is assigned the lowest rank = 1.
- Data observation with biggest value is assigned the highest rank = n (i.e. the total number of obervations in all groups).
- Observations having the same value are assigned a mean of their ranks.
- Having assigned a rank to each data observation, sum all ranks respectively for every group ($\Sigma\gamma$a), ($\Sigma\gamma$b), ($\Sigma\gamma$c), …, ($\Sigma\gamma$z).
- Summed ranks are then compared for difference = H. (Note: The greater the discrepancy between groups the larger the value of H.)

If null hypothesis is correct then $H = 0$ (or near zero). The larger the value of H, the smaller the p-value, which can be read off appropriate statistical tables. P-value expresses the probability of obtaining sum of rank values as discrepant as observed if all treatments were really equivalent.

Table i The z distribution (two-tailed probabilities associated with observations being multiples of the standard deviation in a Normal distribution)

z	0.00	0.01	0.02	0.03	0.04	0.05	0.06	0.07	0.08	0.09
0.00	1.0000	0.9920	0.9840	0.9761	0.9681	0.9601	0.9522	0.9442	0.9362	0.9283
0.10	0.9203	0.9124	0.9045	0.8966	0.8887	0.8808	0.8729	0.8650	0.8572	0.8493
0.20	0.8415	0.8337	0.8259	0.8181	0.8103	0.8206	0.7949	0.7872	0.7795	0.7718
0.30	0.7642	0.7566	0.7490	0.7414	0.7339	0.7263	0.7188	0.7114	0.7039	0.6965
0.40	0.6892	0.6818	0.6745	0.6672	0.6599	0.6527	0.6455	0.6384	0.6312	0.6241
0.50	0.6171	0.6101	0.6031	0.5961	0.5892	0.5823	0.5755	0.5687	0.5619	0.5552
0.60	0.5485	0.5419	0.5353	0.5287	0.5222	0.5157	0.5093	0.5029	0.4965	0.4902
0.70	0.4839	0.4777	0.4715	0.4654	0.4593	0.4533	0.4473	0.4413	0.4354	0.4295
0.80	0.4337	0.4179	0.4122	0.4065	0.4009	0.3953	0.3898	0.3843	0.3789	0.3735
0.90	0.3681	0.3628	0.3576	0.3524	0.3472	0.3421	0.3371	0.3320	0.3271	0.3222
1.00	0.3173	0.3125	0.3077	0.3030	0.2983	0.2837	0.2891	0.2846	0.2801	0.2757
1.10	0.2713	0.2670	0.2627	0.2585	0.2543	0.2501	0.2460	0.2420	0.2380	0.2340
1.20	0.2301	0.2263	0.2225	0.2187	0.2150	0.2113	0.2077	0.2041	0.2005	0.1971
1.30	0.1936	0.1902	0.1868	0.1835	0.1802	0.1770	0.1738	0.1707	0.1676	0.1645
1.40	0.1615	0.1585	0.1556	0.1527	0.1499	0.1471	0.1443	0.1416	0.1389	0.1362
1.50	0.1336	0.1310	0.1285	0.1260	0.1236	0.1211	0.1188	0.1164	0.1141	0.1118
1.60	0.1096	0.1074	0.1052	0.1031	0.1010	0.0989	0.0969	0.0949	0.0930	0.0910
1.70	0.0891	0.0873	0.0854	0.0836	0.0819	0.0801	0.0784	0.0767	0.0751	0.0735
1.80	0.0719	0.0703	0.0688	0.0672	0.0658	0.0643	0.0629	0.0615	0.0601	0.0588
1.90	0.0574	0.0561	0.0549	0.0536	0.0524	0.0512	0.0500	0.0488	0.0477	0.0466
2.00	0.0455	0.0444	0.0434	0.0424	0.0414	0.0404	0.0394	0.0385	0.0375	0.0366
2.10	0.0357	0.0349	0.0340	0.0332	0.0324	0.0316	0.0308	0.0300	0.0293	0.0285
2.20	0.0278	0.0271	0.0264	0.0257	0.0251	0.0244	0.0238	0.0232	0.0226	0.0220
2.30	0.0214	0.0209	0.0203	0.0198	0.0193	0.0188	0.0183	0.0178	0.0173	0.0168
2.40	0.0164	0.0160	0.0155	0.0151	0.0147	0.0143	0.0139	0.0135	0.0131	0.0128
2.50	0.0124	0.0121	0.0117	0.0114	0.0111	0.0108	0.0105	0.0102	0.0099	0.0096
2.60	0.0093	0.0091	0.0088	0.0085	0.0083	0.0080	0.0078	0.0076	0.0074	0.0071
2.70	0.0069	0.0067	0.0065	0.0063	0.0061	0.0060	0.0058	0.0056	0.0054	0.0053
2.80	0.0051	0.0050	0.0048	0.0047	0.0045	0.0044	0.0042	0.0041	0.0040	0.0039
2.90	0.0037	0.0036	0.0035	0.0034	0.0033	0.0032	0.0031	0.0030	0.0029	0.0028
3.00	0.0027	0.0026	0.0025	0.0024	0.0024	0.0023	0.0022	0.0021	0.0021	0.0020

Table ii Distribution of *t* (two-tailed)

df	0.5	0.1	0.05	0.02	0.01	0.001
1	1.000	6.314	12.706	31.821	63.657	636.619
2	0.816	2.920	4.303	6.965	9.925	31.598
3	0.765	2.353	3.182	4.541	5.841	12.941
4	0.741	2.132	2.776	3.747	4.604	8.610
5	0.727	2.015	2.571	3.365	4.032	6.859
6	0.718	1.943	2.447	3.143	3.707	5.959
7	0.711	1.895	2.365	2.998	3.499	5.405
8	0.706	1.860	2.306	2.896	3.355	5.041
9	0.703	1.833	2.262	2.821	3.250	4.781
10	0.700	1.812	2.228	2.764	3.169	4.587
11	0.697	1.796	2.201	2.718	3.106	4.437
12	0.695	1.782	2.179	2.681	3.055	4.318
13	0.694	1.771	2.160	2.650	3.012	4.221
14	0.692	1.761	2.145	2.624	2.977	4.140
15	0.691	1.753	2.131	2.602	2.947	4.073
16	0.690	1.746	2.120	2.583	2.921	4.015
17	0.689	1.740	2.110	2.567	2.898	3.965
18	0.688	1.734	2.101	2.552	2.878	3.922
19	0.688	1.729	2.093	2.539	2.861	3.883
20	0.687	1.725	2.086	2.528	2.845	3.850
21	0.686	1.721	2.080	2.518	2.831	3.819
22	0.686	1.717	2.074	2.508	2.819	3.792
23	0.685	1.714	2.069	2.500	2.807	3.767
24	0.685	1.711	2.064	2.492	2.797	3.745
25	0.684	1.708	2.060	2.485	2.787	3.725
26	0.684	1.706	2.056	2.479	2.779	3.707
27	0.684	1.703	2.052	2.473	2.771	3.690
28	0.683	1.701	2.048	2.467	2.763	3.674
29	0.683	1.699	2.045	2.462	2.756	3.659
30	0.683	1.697	2.042	2.457	2.750	3.646
	0.674	1.645	1.960	2.326	2.576	3.291

Table iii The χ^2 distribution

df	0.2	0.1	0.05	0.04	0.03	0.02	0.01	0.001
1	1.64	2.71	3.84	4.22	4.71	5.41	6.63	10.83
2	3.22	4.61	5.99	6.44	7.01	7.82	9.21	13.82
3	4.64	6.25	7.81	8.31	8.95	9.84	11.34	16.27
4	5.99	7.78	9.49	10.03	10.71	11.67	13.28	18.47
5	7.29	9.24	11.07	11.64	12.37	13.39	15.09	20.52
6	8.56	10.64	12.59	13.20	13.97	15.03	16.81	22.46
7	9.80	12.02	14.07	14.70	15.51	16.62	18.48	24.32
8	11.03	13.36	15.51	16.17	17.01	18.17	20.09	26.13
9	12.24	14.68	16.92	17.61	18.48	19.68	21.67	27.88
10	13.44	15.99	18.31	19.02	19.92	21.16	23.21	29.59
11	14.63	17.28	19.68	20.41	21.34	22.62	24.73	31.26
12	15.81	18.55	21.03	21.79	22.74	24.05	26.22	32.91
13	16.98	19.81	22.36	23.14	24.12	25.47	27.69	34.53
14	18.15	21.06	23.68	24.49	25.49	26.87	29.14	36.12
15	19.31	22.31	25.00	25.82	26.85	28.26	30.58	37.70
16	20.47	23.54	26.30	27.14	28.19	29.63	32.00	39.25
17	21.61	24.77	27.59	28.45	29.52	31.00	33.41	40.79
18	22.76	25.99	28.87	29.75	30.84	32.35	34.81	42.31
19	23.90	27.20	30.14	31.04	32.16	33.69	36.19	43.82
20	25.04	28.41	31.41	32.32	33.46	35.02	37.57	45.32
21	26.17	29.61	32.67	33.60	34.75	36.34	38.91	47.00
22	27.30	30.81	33.92	34.87	36.04	37.65	40.32	48.41
23	28.43	32.01	35.18	36.13	37.33	38.97	41.61	49.81
24	29.55	33.19	36.41	37.39	38.62	40.26	43.02	51.22
25	30.67	34.38	37.65	38.65	39.88	41.55	44.30	52.63
26	31.79	35.56	38.88	39.88	41.14	42.84	45.65	54.03
27	32.91	36.74	40.12	41.14	42.40	44.13	47.00	55.44
28	34.03	37.92	41.35	42.37	43.66	45.42	48.29	56.84
29	35.14	39.09	42.56	43.60	44.92	46.71	49.58	58.25
30	36.25	40.25	43.78	44.83	46.15	47.97	50.87	59.66

Relevant study design issues

2

Hierarchy of evidence

Medical evidence can be obtained from many sources, all of which vary in quality depending on the methods used in establishing them. Naturally, studies that stringently adhere to scientific research principles are given more credence than studies with more relaxed or anecdotal methodologies. Figure 2.1 illustrates the widely accepted hierarchy of the research methodologies.

It must be said, however, that the information obtained from all types of studies has value in that it adds to the general pool of knowledge, and that the less-esteemed study types often form the basis for further research where more robust scientific methods are employed.

Types of studies of study designs

Strengths and weaknesses of various study designs

The various types of studies have their respective advantages and disadvantages, and this area is often exploited in critical appraisal examinations! Table 2.1 highlights some of these attributes.

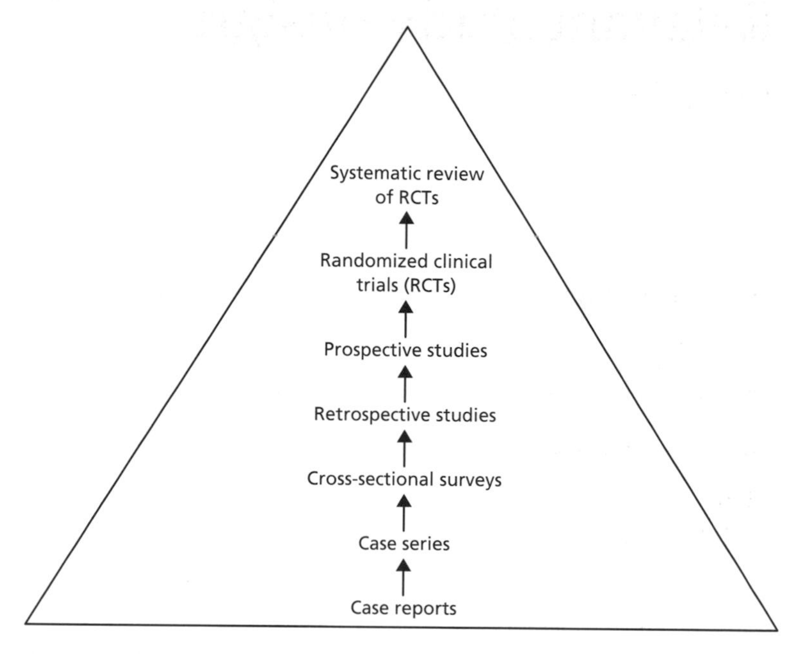

Figure 2.1 Hierarchy of evidence.

Table 2.1 Comparing design strengths and weaknesses

Parameter	Cross-sectional surveys	Case-control studies	Prospective cohort studies	RCTs
Cost	Low	Low	High	High
Set-up	Quick and easy	Quick and easy	Complex	Complex
Recall bias	Low	High	Low	Low
Rare diseases	Impractical	Practical	Impractical	Practical
Rare exposures	Impractical	Disadvantage	Advantage	Deliberate
Long disease course	NA	Advantage	Disadvantage	NA
Diseases with latency	NA	Advantage	Disadvantage	NA
Follow-up period	None	Short	Long	Specified
Attrition rate	NA	Low	High	Moderate
Estimate incidence	NA	Poor	Good	NA
Estimate prognosis	NA	Fair	Good	NA
Examine several possible risks	NA	Good	Impractical	Impractical
Examine several possible outcomes	NA	Impractical	Good	NA
Inference to target population	Strong	Less strong	Strong	Strong

RCTs = randomized clinical trials; NA = not applicable.

The selection process

The process of selection of individuals for participation in a study occurs according to a series of logical steps, before the start of the study. The different stages of the selection process are illustrated in Figure 2.2 in the context of a randomized clinical trial (RCT) study.

Confounding factors

A 'confounding factor' is any factor associated with both the variable(s) of interest and the outcome of a study. It is often an unrecognized or even unmeasured factor that can adversely influence any observations we may make about the relationship between variable(s) and outcome in a study. The presence of confounding factors can therefore weaken the validity of the results obtained from a study.

Unlike other sources of bias in a study, confounding is not created by some overt mistake or other made by the investigators, but arises from real life relationships that already exist between the variables and outcomes under consideration.

In other words, a confounding factor is an intrinsic source of error within an observational study or survey. No such study can ever be entirely free of confounding factors, as many may even be unknown to the researchers. However, efforts to counteract any identified potential confounding factors should start right at the beginning of a study, that is, at the study design stage.

The strength of RCTs lies in the fact that they are free of baseline confounding factors due to the process of randomization. Complete blinding also ensures that there are no subsequent confounding factors during the trial process. (See later chapters.)

EXAMPLE

In a case-control study aiming to examine possible links between alcohol dependence and cerebrovascular disease, 100 subjects known to have cerebrovascular disease (cases) were selected into the study along with 100 subjects known *not* to have cerebrovascular disease. The intent of the researchers was to compare both groups to see which would have a larger proportion of alcoholic subjects present.

In this particular case-control study, cigarette smoking would very likely be a potential confounding factor. This is because cigarette smoking causes cerebrovascular disease and is also common among people with

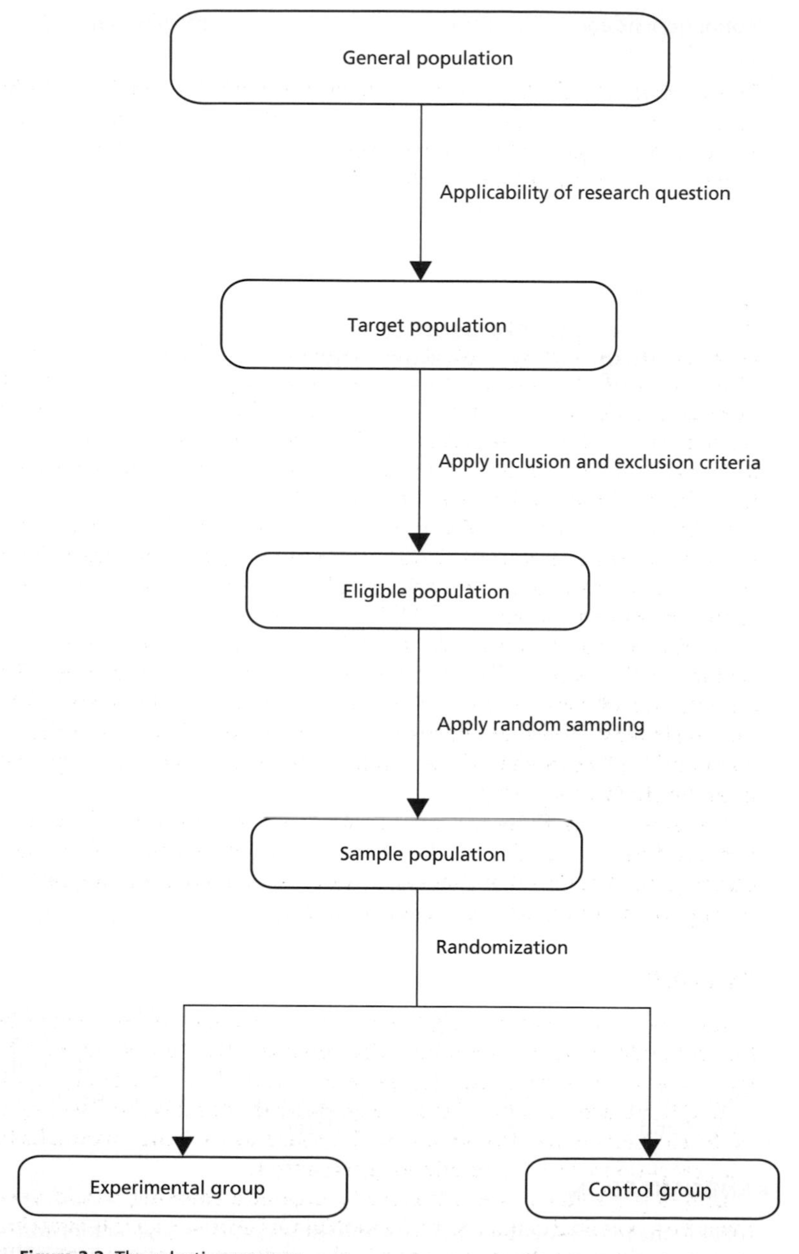

Figure 2.2 The selection process.

alcohol dependence. Therefore, even if the alcoholic group was found to have a higher cerebrovascular disease rate, it would be impossible to know whether this was truly due to alcohol dependence or due to the fact that they happened to smoke more than the control subjects.

Therefore, any observed relationship between alcohol dependence and cerebrovascular disease in such a study becomes less valid unless cigarette smoking is addressed properly as a confounding factor by the researchers.

Measures commonly used to counteract confounding – at the design stage

MATCHING

Here, control subjects are selected based on certain characteristics (usually potential confounding factors) they have in common with experimental subjects. This is done in order that any identified experimental group confounding factors can also be replicated in the control group. Therefore in the example described above, confounding presented by case subjects who smoke can be potentially neutralized by recruiting an equal number of control subjects who also smoke.

When matching, the ideal procedure is to create a control group matched with case subjects on a small number of pertinent criteria. This is because over-matching of subjects can lead to the creation of an *artificial* control population that is less realistic and less representative of the target population.

RESTRICTION

Here, the introduction of confounding into a study is obviated altogether. This is commonly done by use of inclusion and exclusion criteria when selecting participants for a study. As with the example above, if all subjects (experimental and control) with a history of smoking were banned from the study, smoking as a confounding factor would be eliminated altogether. However, over-restriction of subjects should be avoided as this can create sample populations that are far-removed from the real state of things in the target population. Restriction, therefore, has to be justified and based on a set of relevant criteria.

RANDOMIZATION

Probably the most potent method of addressing confounding factors, randomization is used in special type of studies called 'randomized clinical trials' (RCTs). The randomization process (i.e. fixed randomization) ensures that all subjects entering into a study have an equal chance of being allocated to any group within the study. As a result, the presence of confounding factors becomes equally likely in the experimental and control groups. There are a variety of schedules commonly used in the randomization process and details of these should be stated in study reports.

Randomization is discussed in more detail in the clinical trials chapter.

Measures commonly used to counteract confounding – at the stage of result analysis

DATA STRATIFICATION

This describes a technique of separating all collected data by a confounding factor during the stage of result analysis. Therefore, in the example described above, data on all case and control subjects that smoke can be set apart from the data on non-smoking subjects. The effects of confounding factors usually become apparent after stratification.

A high index of suspicion and clinical judgement are often necessary to know the appropriate confounding factors by which to stratify the data in a study.

STATISTICAL MODELLING

These are complex statistical manoeuvres that are often employed to examine the exact nature of the relationship between the variable(s) and the outcomes of a study as well as to explore the impact that any other confounding factors or relationships may have had on the study results. With statistical modelling, therefore, researchers can address the imperfections that inevitably occur in all studies. (See correlation and regression methods discussed in the statistics chapter.)

Bias

Bias is the term that is used to describe the presence of systematic error in a study. A systematic error is an error that does not occur by chance. The presence of bias at any stage of a study (e.g. design, data collection or analysis stage) undermines the validity of study results and the conclusions that can be drawn from them. Bias results from overt mistakes made by investigators. The following describe some famous types of bias.

Observer bias

Observer bias occurs whenever subjective factors within an assessor systematically affect the way observations are scored or recorded. For example, a doctor who has a personal preference for 'Treatment A' may unconsciously be scoring patients on Treatment A more favourably than patients on 'Treatment B' whilst also searching for undesirable side-effects with more vigour with Treatment B subjects than with Treatment A subjects. Such is the human nature.

BLIND ASSESSMENT OF OUTCOME

A common method of counteracting observer bias is through the process of 'blinding'. Blinding ensures that the assessors remain unaware of the groups to which subjects belong. When this information is concealed from the:

- Subjects: single-blind.
- Subjects and clinicians/Assessors: double-blind.
- Subjects and clinicians/assessors, and result analyst: triple-blind (this is a relatively new term).

Asking subjects and assessors after the study about what groups they believe subjects had belonged to can examine the integrity of the blinding process put in place during a study. Any flaws in the blinding process should be suspected if either the subjects or assessors systematically 'get it right'.

STRUCTURED INTERVIEWS

Structured interviews used by assessors when gathering data can be incorporated in the study design to address the element of subjectivity on the part of the assessors, thereby reducing the chance of observer bias in a study.

MULTIPLE ASSESSORS

The use of several assessors in a study may also minimize the impact that any one assessor may have as a source of bias, although this can be rendered ineffective if all assessors are subject to the same biased expectations. The use of multiple assessors does however, introduce another problem, which is to do with the uniformity of their methods. In order to ensure uniformity, all assessors may be similarly pre-trained and pre-tested on the rating of observations. (See inter-rater reliability.)

Selection bias

Selection bias is said to occur whenever a characteristic associated with the variable(s) or outcome of a study affects the very probability of being selected for participation in that study. When it occurs, selection bias often results in study populations comprising participants who are not wholly representative of the target population. Clearly, selection bias can undermine any meaningful inferences that may be drawn from study results.

Ideally, study participants should be randomly selected from the eligible population according to a pre-determined protocol ('random sampling'), but the requirement of obtaining informed patient consent makes this impossible in practice.

SIMPLE RANDOM SAMPLING

Participants are randomly selected from a defined eligible population by use of methods such as computer-generated random numbers. All individuals in the eligible population therefore have an equal probability of being selected for study participation.

SYSTEMATIC SAMPLING

With this commonly used method, every *n*th subject is selected from the population. However, the first subject (e.g. from the list) should be picked by a purely random method. Following this, every *n*th subsequent subject can then be selected thereafter.

STRATIFIED RANDOM SAMPLING

This method is useful for cases where the representation of certain population subsets (*strata*) are deemed necessary in a study (e.g. certain age groups). Therefore, after dividing the eligible population into the desired strata, random sampling is then applied to each stratum in turn, resulting in a sample with each stratum being represented proportionately.

MULTISTAGE RANDOM SAMPLING

With this method, random sampling is performed at two or more stages in the selection process. For example, in selecting school children for an 'attitude-towards-bullying' survey, random sampling of schools may initially be performed in the local area. This can then be followed in the second stage by a random selection of pupils from the already selected schools.

CLUSTER SAMPLING

A form of random sampling that is somewhat similar to multistage sampling. However, after the initial random sampling of centres at the first stage, no further random selection is done with cluster sampling. Instead, all the subjects in these chosen centres are selected for participation. In effect, random sampling is only applied to the centres, creating clusters of subjects.

Prevalence bias

This type of bias is said to occur when sample subjects are chosen exclusively from a specialized setting containing people with a 'special' form of the disorder of interest. Naturally, such subjects would not be entirely representative of all those at risk in the target population.

Such potent samples tend to comprise subjects with more chronic or more severe forms of disorder, undermining the validity of any inferences that can be drawn to the rest of the target population.

EXAMPLE

A randomized clinical trial (RCT) is conducted to examine the efficacy of an educational self-help leaflet (as an adjunct to dietary advice) in the initial treatment for obesity. In this study, 50 obese subjects selected from a *specialist obesity clinic population* were randomized to receive either dietary advice alone or dietary advice along with a self-help leaflet.

Whatever the outcome, results from this study can only be narrowly generalized because the subjects chosen for the study were likely to be systematically different from most obese people in the general population.

Recall bias

The ability to recall past events accurately varies from person to person, and this is a particular problem in retrospective studies where differences in recall abilities are often observed between people with disorder and people without disorder. These differences occur because individuals with disorder are more likely than healthy control subjects to remember real or perceived exposures to risk factors in the past. (Note: The converse is true with certain disorders, e.g. Alzheimer's disease, where recall abilities are reduced as part and parcel of the clinical syndrome.)

When compared with healthy control subjects, individuals with disorder are likely to have had more frequent contacts with healthcare providers. Such frequent contacts can result in increased health awareness and greater understanding of the disease process, etc. in these experimental subjects.

Furthermore, 'response priming' can occur in a study with subjects who have chronic conditions, and results from the countless number of similar enquiries made by clinicians in the past. Although this phenomenon is not, strictly speaking, a part of recall bias, it is partly responsible for the observation that those with a chronic disorder often make better historians.

The impact of recall bias in a study can be reduced with the use of objective instruments and methods in the gathering or corroboration of information wherever applicable, for example structured interviews, hospital records, social service records, employment records, etc. Other studies may recruit people with another (though similar) disorder as control subjects so as to reduce the impact of recall bias.

EXAMPLE

One hundred children diagnosed with autism were recruited into a retrospective case-control study examining a possible relationship between childhood autism and intra-uterine exposure to influenza virus.

The possible effect of increased health awareness that generally results from parenting an autistic child and a variety of other factors prompted researchers in this study to anticipate that the mothers of autistic children may recall 'flu-like illnesses during pregnancy more frequently than the mothers of healthy children. Other factors included the likelihood that mothers of autistic children would have had more frequent contacts with health workers in the past or that they would have been asked about gestational illnesses more often in the past compared to the mothers of healthy children.

Therefore, in order to address recall bias, 100 children attending the same hospital and diagnosed with attention deficit disorder (ADHD) were used as control subjects in the study.

Information bias

Information bias arises from systematic misclassification of data in a study. Information bias is a not-infrequently occurring form of bias that can make a complete nonsense of study results. It can arise in a study from a variety of sources, including:

- A poor theoretical understanding of the disorder of interest or its associated factors leading to misdiagnosis and misclassification of subjects.

- Carelessness such as mistakes made when measuring or classifying data resulting in the wrongful classification of subjects' disease status or exposure status.
- Use of instruments with poor validity. Here, the variable intended for measurement may not be measured accurately or measured at all because of an invalid or wrongly applied instrument.
- Subject-related factors, such as the inaccurate reporting of symptoms, social desirability, faking good, faking bad, etc. (See the chapter on cross-sectional surveys.)

Critical appraisal of studies on diagnostic tests

3

Introduction

In this chapter, we consider a systematic approach to determining the validity of a test, that is, how good a test is at measuring what it is supposed to measure as well as general approach to critically appraising research papers reporting on screening or diagnostic test validity. These papers are often featured in critical appraisal examinations.

Critical appraisal of studies about diagnostic or screening tests:

- Is the study design methodologically sound?
- How does the test perform?
- How do the results affect the care of my patients?

Is the study design methodologically sound?

The following are the main considerations when appraising a study that has been conducted to examine the validity of a diagnostic test or a screening test.

- Ensure that the participants in the study include those with the disorder and those without the disorder being tested for. This is a crucial methodological issue that is necessary when assessing the validity of a new test in order to measure the error rate of the test *vis-à-vis* false positive and false negative rates.

- Ensure that the participants in the study include individuals with all the clinically important forms or stages of disease. A full representation of the various forms and stages of the disease ensures that any reported observations on test performance can be truly applicable to the majority (if not all) of those at risk. Any methodological shortcomings on this equally crucial methodological issue should be stated in the study report.
- Ensure that along with the new test, a gold standard test was also applied to *all* the participants in the study. Study authors should also justify the choice of the gold standard test. Whenever a questionable test is used as a gold standard test, the new test that is under examination cannot but also have questionable validity.
- Ensure that the gold standard test was applied independently of the new test. The policy of applying both experimental and the gold standard tests independently of each other in every study subject guards against any possible carry-over of effects from one test application to the other. Independent testing also guards against the 'work-up bias' that occurs when tests are carried out in rapid succession in the same individual. Here, the process of having applied one test immediately before applying another significantly influences the responses obtained with the latter test.
- Ensure that the clinicians were blind to new test results when applying gold standard test and vice versa. Clearly, this is in order to guard against observer bias on the part of the researchers.
- Ensure that the test validation process described above was conducted on subjects different from those on whom the test was initially developed, that is, in the early test development stages.

How does the test perform?

The validity of a test, that is, how good a test is at doing its job, forms the basis of how much the test can be trusted and, therefore, the clinical usefulness of that test. Measuring the performance of such a test in comparison with a gold standard is regarded as the best way of assessing test validity. The indices of test performance or test validity commonly measured are: sensitivity, specificity, likelihood ratios, negative and positive predictive values.

Sensitivity

	Gold standard		
Test	Disease	Well	Total
Positive	A	B	A + B
Negative	C	D	C + D
Total	A + C	B + D	A + B + C + D

Sensitivity = A/(A + C)

The sensitivity of a test is defined as any of the following:

- Proportion of true positives correctly identified by a test, or
- Proportion of patients with disease (confirmed by a gold standard) testing positive, or
- Ability of test to correctly identify true positives, or
- The chance of a positive test result given a disease.

A worked example:

	Gold standard		
Test	Disease	Well	Total
Positive	80	40	120
Negative	20	60	80
Total	100	100	200

Sensitivity = A/(A + C)
= 80/100
= 0.8

A test with a sensitivity of 0.8 will always identify 80% of true cases correctly.

Specificity

	Gold standard		
Test	Disease	Well	Total
Positive	A	B	A + B
Negative	C	D	C + D
Total	A + C	B + D	A + B + C + D

Specificity = D/(B + D)

The specificity of a test can be defined as any of the following:

- Proportion of true negatives correctly identified by a test, or
- Proportion of patients without disease (confirmed by gold standard) testing negative, or
- Ability of test to correctly identify true negatives, or
- The chance of a negative test result given no disease.

A worked example:

	Gold standard		
Test	Disease	Well	Total
Positive	80	40	120
Negative	20	60	80
Total	100	100	200

Specificity = D/(B + D)
= 60/100
= 0.6

A test with a specificity of 0.6 will always identify 60% of true non-cases correctly.

About sensitivity and specificity

Like the introvert and extrovert personality traits within an individual, the sensitivity and specificity of a test exist in an inverse relationship – like a seesaw. Furthermore, unless a test is completely redesigned, the sensitivity and specificity values for that test do not change. They remain constant regardless of the setting in which the test is being used and regardless of the prevalence of the variable being tested for.

Tests with continuous results

In contrast to binary (*positive/negative*) test result categories, many tests produce results of a continuous numerical nature. This is true of several biochemical tests and questionnaire tests used in clinical practice. Tests with hybrid result categories are also common in clinical practice where a particular value on a numerical scale is chosen as a cut-off point below which the test is deemed negative and above which the test is deemed positive or vice versa. Whatever the formats that test results exist in, the test sensitivity and specificity values remain constant.

How are test cut-off points determined?

When designing a new test, the sensitivity and specificity values to be possessed by that test are major considerations. As already stated, however, sensitivity and specificity values of a test have an inverse relationship. As one improves, the other deteriorates as one varies the cut-off point of the test.

Theoretically, the most desirable balance between the values of sensitivity and specificity to be possessed by a test can be determined by a lengthy procedure that involves measuring the sensitivity and specificity values at different cut-off points using a gold standard as reference. The test cut-off point responsible for producing the best attainable sensitivity–specificity compromise then becomes the declared theoretical cut-off point of that test (Table 3.1).

Table 3.1 Finding the best sensitivity and specificity trade-off using the MMSE test as an illustration

Cut-off	Sensitivity	Specificity
1	0.10	0.90
2	0.12	0.98
3	0.13	0.97
4	0.15	0.96
5	0.18	0.95
6	0.21	0.94
7	0.25	0.92
8	0.29	0.90
9	0.33	0.89
10	0.39	0.84
11	0.44	0.81
12	0.51	0.79
18	0.53	0.77
24	0.75	0.75
25	0.79	0.61
26	0.84	0.42
27	0.89	0.32
28	0.92	0.23
29	0.96	0.18
30	0.99	0.13

The sensitivity and specificity values obtained for these respective cut-off points can also be presented graphically presented on a receiver operating characteristic (ROC) curve, such as Figure 3.1. The closest point on the ROC curve to the ideal state represents the best sensitivity–specificity compromise attainable by the test. See Figure 3.2.

The total area under the ROC curve (AUC) of a test represents the probability of that test correctly identifying true positives and true negatives,

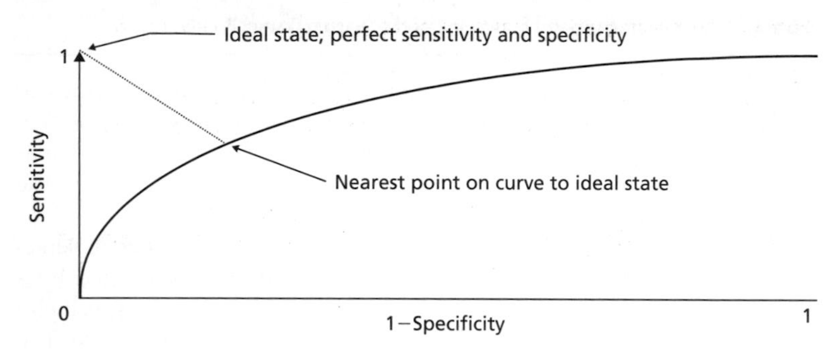

Figure 3.1 The receiver operating characteristic (ROC) plot.

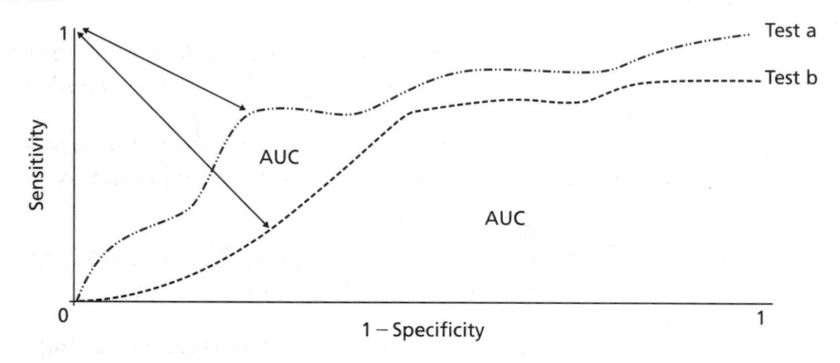

Figure 3.2 Comparison of different tests re-performance using the ROC curve.

that is, test accuracy. As shown in Figure 3.2, the AUC of similar tests can be directly compared on the ROC curve. Here, 'Test a' performs better than 'Test b'.

In certain clinical situations, however, the cut-off point of a test can sometimes be purposely set at another point on the ROC curve away from the so described best compromise cut-off point. This is usually done in order to make the test more clinically useful because changing the cut-off point at which a test operates will change the sensitivity and specificity values of that test (Table 3.2).

The impact of such a modification of test cut-off point is explored in the clinical examples below.

EXAMPLE 1

On the Mini-Mental State Examination (MMSE) screening test, a score of 24 or less, out of a possible total of 30 is taken as being indicative of

Table 3.2 The meaning of (1 – sensitivity) and (1 – specificity) in plain English

Sensitivity: True positive rate *'How good at identifying disease'*	(1 – specificity): False positive rate *'Mistake rate when identifying normality'*
(1 – sensitivity): False negative rate *'Mistake rate when identifying disease'*	Specificity: True negative rate *'How good at identifying normality'*

a possible dementia diagnosis, that is, a cut-off point of 24/30. However, if the MMSE test cut-off point were arbitrarily set at 4/30, three interesting things would happen:

- Many potential dementia cases would be missed, i.e. low sensitivity.
- Virtually no well people would be wrongly identified as possible dementia cases, that is, high specificity.
- A positive result (i.e. four or less) in this high specificity–low sensitivity version of the MMSE test would rule in a strong possibility of dementia.

Conversely, if the MMSE test cut-off point were arbitrarily set at 29/30, three contrasting but equally interesting things would happen:

- Virtually no possible dementia cases would be missed, that is, high sensitivity.
- Many well people would be wrongly identified as possible dementia cases, that is, low specificity.
- A negative result (i.e. 30) in this high sensitivity–low specificity version of the MMSE test would rule out any possible dementia.

EXAMPLE 2

You have been asked by your Health Authority to select one of two tests that would be used as a screening tool for early carcinoma of the cervix in your community. Test A is associated with a sensitivity of 0.99 and a specificity of 0.6. Test B, on the other hand, is associated with a sensitivity of 0.85 and a specificity of 0.95.

Implications of use of Test A as a screening tool:

- Test A would correctly identify about 99% of all true early cervical cancer cases, which suggests a low theshold for detecting cervical cancer. Therefore, cancerous cervical changes are rarely missed (i.e. a low false negative rate). This is just as well. The cost of a false negative diagnosis with cervical carcinoma can be disasterous or even fatal.

- However, the use of Test A would also mean that up to 40% of normal cases would be falsely diagnosed as being cancerous (i.e. a high false positive rate). Although these false positive smears can ultimately be declared non-cancerous after further investigation, the cost of false positive screen results for these patients would be a few weeks of needless anxiety, along with the inconvenience of further investigations, not to mention the added financial cost.

Implications of use of Test B as a screening tool:

- Test B would correctly identify about 85% of cases, missing about 15% of early cervical cancer cases. A 15% miss rate when screening for cervical cancer clearly makes Test B less clinically desirable than Test A. This is despite the fact that Test B would rarely identify normal cases incorrectly as being cancerous (5%) because of a high 95% specificity.

Obviously, in this clinical scenario the cost of a false negative diagnosis, that is, missed early carcinoma, is far greater than the cost of false positive diagnosis, that is, patient inconvenience, anxiety and additional financial costs. The higher sensitivity and lower specificity figures possessed by Test A make it a more clinically valuable test, likely to save many more lives than Test B.

Positive predictive value

	Gold standard		
Test	Disease	Well	Total
Positive	A	B	A + B
Negative	C	D	C + D
Total	A + C	B + D	A + B + C + D

Positive predictive value (PPV) = A/(A + B)

The positive predictive value (PPV) of a test is defined as the:

- Proportion of positive test results for which disease is confirmed, or
- Probability that the patient is a true positive (having disease), having tested positive, or
- The chance of disease given a positive result.

A worked example:

Gold standard			
Test	Disease	Well	Total
Positive	80	40	120
Negative	20	60	80
Total	100	100	200

PPV = A/(A + B)
= 80/120
= 0.67

A PPV of 0.67 means that after a positive test result, there is a 67% chance of having the disease.

Negative predictive value

Gold standard			
Test	Disease	Well	Total
Positive	A	B	A + B
Negative	C	D	C + D
Total	A + C	B + D	A + B + C + D

Negative predictive value = D/(C + D)

The negative predictive value (NPV) of a test is defined as the:

- Proportion of negative test results for which disease is absent, or
- Probability that the patient is a true negative (without disease), having tested negative, or
- The chance of no disease given a negative result.

A worked example:

Gold standard			
Test	Disease	Well	Total
Positive	80	40	120
Negative	20	60	80
Total	100	100	200

NPV = D/(C + D)
= 60/80
= 0.75

An NPV of 0.75 means that after a negative result, there is a 75% chance of not having the disease.

As discussed earlier, the sensitivity and specificity of a test are unaffected by prevalence. In contrast, the PPV and NPV of a test are affected by prevalence. The relationship between prevalence and both predictive values (Figure 3.3) can be summarized as follows:

- The PPV of a test is higher if the test is applied in a high-prevalence setting, such as an inpatient ward, than if applied in a low-prevalence setting, like the general community. This is because in a high-prevalence setting a test simply has a higher chance of coming into contact with true cases than non-cases and hence a greater chance of a true-positive than a false-positive result.
- Conversely, in a low-prevalence setting, a test has a higher chance of coming into contact with non-cases than true cases and hence a greater chance of a false-positive than a true-positive result.
- Similarly, the NPV of a test is higher if the test is applied in a low-prevalence setting, such as in the community, than if applied in a high-prevalence setting, such as an inpatient ward.

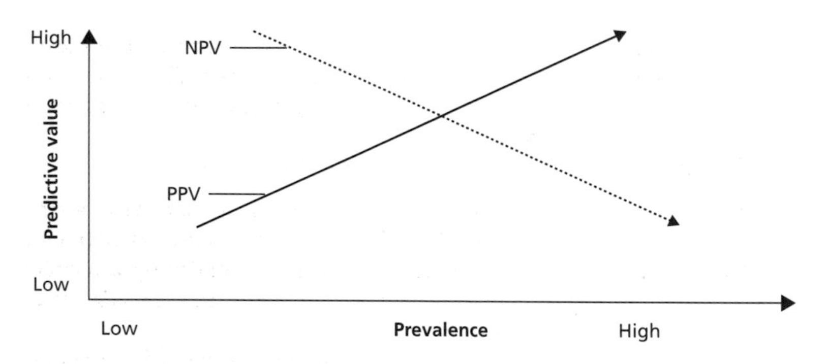

Figure 3.3 Relationship between prevalence and predictive values. NPV = negative predictive value; PPV = positive predictive value.

Other bits and pieces about test validity

	Gold standard		
Test	Disease	Well	Total
Positive	A	B	A + B
Negative	C	D	C + D
Total	A + C	B + D	A + B + C + D

Prevalence of disease = (A + C)/(A + B + C + D)
Screen Prevalence = (A + B)/(A + B + C + D)
Accuracy of test = (A + D)/(A + B + C + D)

A typical examination vignette

In a study recently reported in a medical journal, a new questionnaire is designed as a screening tool for alcoholism. In the study, 100 consecutive people (*anybody*) walking through the doors of a large AA centre (*high-prevalence setting*) were screened with the questionnaire. Screening was followed by standardised interviews conducted by a physician (*gold standard*).

The new questionnaire is reported to have performed as follows.

	Physician positive	Physician negative	Total
Questionnaire positive	22	20	42
Questionnaire negative	18	40	58
Total	40	60	100

Having read about the study members of a local patient care group ask you about the performance of the new questionnaire. They also wondered if it was a suitable tool to use in their GP surgeries (*low-prevalence setting*) to screen GP clients for alcoholism.

Regarding the performance of the new questionnaire:

- The specificity of the new questionnaire (0.67) is higher than its sensitivity (0.55). This means that the new questionnaire is better at identifying non-alcoholic people than it is at identifying alcoholic people. This is particularly interesting as the questionnaire was designed to screen for alcoholism!
- Being identified as alcoholic by the questionnaire should not necessarily cause concern because almost half (48%) of such clients would not be alcoholics (PPV = 0.52).
- A 'not-alcoholic' result should reassure the clinician because 69% of such clients would really be non-alcoholic (NPV = 0.69).

With regard to the suitability of the test for use in a GP practice, that is, a low-prevalence setting:

- The sensitivity of the questionnaire (0.55) would be unchanged, that is, 45% of alcoholic GP clients would go undetected.
- The specificity of the questionnaire (0.67) would be unchanged, that is, 33% of 'non-alcoholic' GP clients would be misidentified as having alcohol problems.

- The PPV of the questionnaire (0.52) would deteriorate, that is, of those clients identified as alcoholic even less than 52% would really have alcohol problems.
- The NPV of the questionnaire (0.69) would improve, that is, of those clients screened as not alcoholic even more than 69% would truly have no such problems.

In summary, the questionnaire is not a particularly useful tool for screening for alcoholism and would be even less effective if applied to a GP client population.

Likelihood ratios

By combining the sensitivity and specificity values of a test, a more versatile and readily applicable measure of test validity may be derived. This measure, called a 'likelihood ratio' (LR), can be calculated for every possible result category of a test. The LR of a given test result is defined as the probability of that test result being seen in an individual with disorder relative to it being seen in an unaffected individual.

In a test with positive and negative (*binary*) result categories, an LR can be calculated for each category.

LIKELIHOOD RATIO FOR POSITIVE RESULT

$$\text{LR positive} = \text{sensitivity}/(1 - \text{specificity})$$

(True-positive rate/False-positive rate)

This ratio describes the likelihood of having a disease, as opposed to not having the disease, having tested positive for it. 'LR+ve' gives clinicians an estimate of the amount by which a positive test result increases the probability of actually having the disease that was tested for. For example, if the LR for a positive Heaf test result is 10, it means that Mr Smith would be ten times more likely to have tuberculosis than not, if he tests positive.

LIKELIHOOD RATIO FOR NEGATIVE RESULT

$$\text{LR negative} = (1 - \text{sensitivity})/\text{specificity}$$

(False-negative rate/True-negative rate)

This ratio describes the likelihood of having a disease as opposed to not having that disease having tested negative for it. 'LR−ve' gives clinicians an estimate of the amount by which a negative test result decreases the probability of having the disease that was tested for.

For example, if the LR for a negative Heaf test result is 0.04, it means that Mr Smith would be 0.04 times more likely (25 times less likely) to have tuberculosis than to be tuberculosis-free, if he tests negative.

WHY LIKELIHOOD RATIOS?

First, LRs are derived from the sensitivity and specificity of a test, and they are also unaffected by prevalence. LRs are thus constant, regardless of different disease prevalence in the various settings where that test may be applied.

Second, LRs are particularly helpful to clinicians because they allow better understanding of test results by suggesting how strongly a positive result indicates disease and how strongly a negative result indicates absence of disease. In other words, LRs indicate how much a test result changes the pre-test probability to a post-test probability of having a disease.

The steps below summarize how the pre-test probability of having a disease can be converted to a post-test probability by use of LRs.

Using likelihood ratios

- Prevalence (A + C)/(A + B + C + D) = pre-test probability.
- Pre-test odds = pre-test probability/(1 − pre-test probability).
- Post-test odds = pre-test odds × LR.
- Post-test probability = post-test odds/(post-test odds + 1).

Relationship between probabilities and odds

'Probability' is defined as the chance of an event occurring. Probability is expressed as a decimal between zero and one.

The 'odds' of an event happening are defined as the probability that the event will occur compared with the probability that the event will not occur:

- Odds = probability/(1 − probability).

(Note: Probability = odds/(odds + 1.)

Likelihood ratios are also used with multi-category or continuous results.

EXAMPLE: USING LRs WITH TESTS THAT HAVE BINARY RESULT CATEGORIES

When the pre-test probability (*prevalence*) of having a disease is known, LRs can be used to calculate the post-test probability of having (or not having) that disease. The following example illustrates how this is done.

A new β4 test is the commonly used screening tool for HIV in a country with a high prevalence of 20%. In its design phase the β4 test was shown to have a sensitivity of 0.99 and a specificity of 0.98. A gentleman named Guy has just received a positive β4 test result for HIV. Understandably distraught, he questions the results and wonders if the test is reliable.

With the HIV prevalence figures and the sensitivity and specificity figures for the β4 test, the doctor reaches the following conclusions that help him to offer accurate advice to his patient:

- Pre-test probability of HIV:

  = 0.2 (20%).

  (There is initially a one in five chance of Guy being HIV positive because he belongs to a population with a 20% prevalence rate.)
- Pre-test odds of HIV:

  = probability/(1 − probability)
  = 0.2/(1 − 0.2)
  = 0.25 (i.e. four to one odds)
- LR for positive result:

  = sensitivity/(1 − specificity)
  = 0.99/0.02
  = 49.5

  (Having tested positive, Guy is now 49.5 times more likely to have than not to have HIV.)
- Post-test odds of HIV:

  = pre-test odds × LR for a positive result
  = 0.25 × 49.5
  = 11 (Odds are now 11 to 1 on)
- Post-test probability:

  = odds/(odds + 1)
  = 11/(11 + 1)
  = 0.92

  (Following his positive β4 test, the chance of Guy being HIV positive is now 92%.)

EXAMPLE: USING LRs WITH TESTS THAT HAVE MULTI-CATEGORY RESULTS

A questionnaire, a new screening tool for post-natal depression, has recently been developed. It scores new mothers on a scale of 1–15 depending on the severity of their symptoms. Mothers can be classified as being 'negative', 'mild positive', 'moderate positive' or 'severe positive' for depression, depending on the score attained on the questionnaire. LRs were established for each result category at the design stage of the test.

Score on questionnaire	Result category	Likelihood ratio
<5	Negative	0.8
5–8	Mild	2.1
9–12	Moderate	7.2
>12	Severe	45

According to the data above, a score of 12 or more on the questionnaire has a particularly high LR of 45, much higher than for a score of 9–12.

Mothers scoring 12 or more in the questionnaire are over six times more likely to be depressed than those scoring between nine and 12 (LR 45 versus 7.2).

Mothers who score between nine and 12 on the questionnaire are only over three times more likely to be depressed than those scoring between five and eight (LR 7.2 versus 2.1) and so on.

The likelihood of having post-natal depression after a negative questionnaire result is 0.8, that is, very unlikely.

As illustrated here, calculating a likelihood ratio for post-natal depression in each of the four result categories, as opposed to just positive and negative categories, allows for more accurate and less restricted intepretation of results by clinicians.

How do the results affect the care of my patients?

This aspect is concerned with how applicable the results of studies on diagnostic tests are to the care of patients and how they may (if at all) change your practice.

- Results on test performance may have implications for your practice if the area of healthcare concerned is directly relevant to the patients in your care.
- A diagnostic test reported as performing highly accurately may not be of much use clinically if the disease being tested for is already easily recognizable, for example the common cold.
- A test may also be of limited use if test results are not likely to alter the management of the disease condition in question.
- Ensure that the subjects in the study of test performance are not essentially different from your patients.

- Test performance results may have urgent implications for screening procedures in cases where early and accurate detection has an impact on morbidity or mortality.
- Resource issues in certain clinical situations may limit widespread use of a proven test.

This is where your clinical judgement based on experience and expertise comes into play.

Critical appraisal of cross-sectional surveys

4

Introduction

Cross-sectional studies are observational types of studies in which the prevalence of a trait or disease condition is measured by snapshot assessments across a given population. Compare this to randomized clinical trials (RCTs), which test hypotheses on the treatment of disease, or prospective and retrospective studies, which test hypotheses on the aetiology of disease. Prevalence and incidence rates are described in more detail in the 'glossary of terms' at the end of the book.

Because subjects are not followed up in time, cross-sectional surveys are poor at measuring the rates of occurrence of new cases of a disease in the population, that is, 'incidence rates' but they can be used to measure prevalence rates of disease.

Types of cross-sectional surveys

Cross-sectional surveys can take any one of several forms, all of which have their own unique sets of advantages and disadvantages.

Surveys involving direct contact with responders

Surveys may involve direct contact with responders, such as telephone surveys or face-to-face interviews. The advantages of these methods are that because researchers are directly involved, more information can be gathered from subjects than with non-contact form filling. This results in more operational flexibility and increased variety of obtained responses.

Probing and clarification of responses can occur on the spot, allowing for increased accuracy of gathered information. Response rates are also generally higher with contact than with non-contact surveys.

The disadvantages of contact surveys are that researchers may inadvertently influence or even stifle responses during direct contact. Direct contact surveys are more expensive and time-consuming to conduct, taking up a lot of researcher time and effort.

Surveys involving no contact with responders

These surveys include self-completed questionnaires (Table 4.1); be it postal or situational, and surveys of records. The advantages with these methods are that they are cheaper and much less time-consuming to undertake. Results are also easier to analyse because of the increased structure that inevitably accompanies such survey responses. In addition, there is less scope for observer bias because responders do not feel the need to be polite to assessors nor do they feel pressurized.

Disadvantages include a lower response rate and less opportunity for responders to express their views as they see fit. The highly structured format of such surveys usually narrows the scope of possible responses.

Surveys with structured and unstructured interview or questionnaire formats

The primary survey aims and survey sample size largely determine the degree of structure to be attached to the format of a survey. Unstructured surveys contain open questions and therefore offer a high degree of flexibility to the responders who are then able to express themselves freely. However, the increased depth and scope provided by this reduced structure causes impossible difficulties when analysing such results, particularly in very large surveys.

Structured surveys are ideal when measuring a finite set of variables and are a blessing when analysing the results of very large surveys. This is because responses from one responder are readily comparable to

Table 4.1 Types of scales used in questionnaire items

Scale / Question	Response format
Binary nominal scale *Do you smoke*?	Yes____ or No____
Multi-category nominal scale *How do you travel to work?*	Car ______ Train ______ Cycle ______ Ferry ______ Other ______
Likert scale *The death penalty should be abolished!*	Strongly agree ___ Agree ___ No opinion ___ Disagree ___ Strongly disagree ___
Visual analogue scale *How would you rate your mood today?*	Suicidal ————————— Perfect
Semantic differential scale *About your doctor?*	Uncaring 0 1 2 3 4 5 Caring Incompetent 0 1 2 3 4 5 Competent Accessible 0 1 2 3 4 5 Inaccessible Dependable 0 1 2 3 4 5 Undependable
Thurstone scale *How many of the following political statements apply to you?* (Note: all items are scored.)	I am concerned about the environment _____ I think environmental issues have too large a profile _____ I have some sympathy with the actions of eco-warriors _____ Global warming needs to be addressed urgently _____ I would give up my car if it makes a difference _____ Alternative energy technology is a big joke! _____ Environmentalists thrive on paranoia _____

those from another responder. However, structured surveys provide information with narrower perspective due to the use of closed questions and this can be a disadvantage.

Semi-structured survey formats

A carefully constructed semi-structured survey draws on the respective strengths of the above contrasting survey formats. Semi-structured surveys contain sections where responses are structured and sections with less structure that allow responders to clarify and elaborate on initial responses and to even raise new issues that have been missed by researchers.

Types of responder-related bias

Volunteer bias

Applies especially to cross-sectional surveys where differences in things such as motivation, socio-economic status and other risk factors are seen to exist between those who choose to participate and those who choose not to participate in a survey. These differences are a major cause of sampling error (i.e. the gathering of unrepresentative information) in a survey. It occurs particularly when the selection process is performed on an invitational basis.

Social desirability

The unconscious tendency of some responders to give socially desirable 'goody-goody' answers. These responders tend to minimize qualities that may be deemed socially undesirable (*'How many times a month do you use recreational cannabis?'*) and they tend to exaggerate their socially desirable qualities (*'How many times a week do you read bedtime stories to your child?'*). Social desirability is a non-deliberate unconscious phenomenon and is related to the personality of the individual.

Deviation

The unconscious tendency of some responders to give socially deviant answers. These subjects are often young rebellious risk-takers who see themselves as leading a lifestyle alternative to the mainstream. Deviation is also an unconscious personality phenomenon.

Faking good

The conscious and deliberate version of *social desirability* where subjects purposely give untrue or exaggerated responses to create a good impression of themselves or of the service for some perceived gains.

Faking bad

The conscious and deliberate version of *deviation* where subjects purposely give untrue or exaggerated responses in return for some perceived gains by making themselves look as bad as possible.

The above types of responder-related bias could be mitigated to an extent in a survey by disguising the real intent of the survey (a dodgy area) or by the inclusion of some seemingly straightforward question items that covertly measure specific personality traits in the respondents.

'Yes'-sayers and 'No'-sayers

Phenomena where subjects have a tendency to always give positive responses (*'yes'-sayers*) or to always give negative responses (*'no'-sayers*). Unlike with the social desirability or deviation responders, here, consistent yes or no responses are given regardless of social norms, and unlike the fakers, these phenomena are wholly unconscious. These responder biases can be identified with the inclusion of contradictory question items.

Positive skew and negative skew

The Likert and visual analogue scale (VAS) equivalents of the yes- and no-saying phenomena. Here, the tendency is to consistently give positive-end or negative-end responses.

End aversion or central tendency bias

A type of responder bias that occurs with Likert or visual analogue scales where responders have an unconscious tendency to avoid extreme categories, thereby essentially constricting the range of possible responses. This bias can be mitigated in a survey by adding extra dummy categories at the ends of a scale in order to preserve the spectrum of genuine responses.

In summary, the critical appraisal of a cross-sectional survey considers:

- **Is survey design methodologically sound?**
- **What do results show?**
- **How do results affect the care of my patients?**

Conducting a cross-sectional survey can be fraught with many potential pitfalls, all of which should ideally be addressed by researchers at the planning stage in order to ensure that the information gathered from a survey is valid and can be generalized to the target population.

Is the survey design methodologically sound?

The issues discussed below are the main considerations when assessing the strengths and weaknesses of cross-sectional survey designs.

Is there a clear statement of aims and a clear description of target population?

A clear statement of research aims and a clear description of the target population are important when reporting a cross-sectional survey. This is because, ultimately, a judgement has to be passed on how well the information gathered from a survey can answer the research question and how applicable survey results are to the target population.

Is the chosen type of survey appropriate?

In the light of the aims of a cross-sectional survey, authors have to justify the reasoning behind the type of survey chosen *vis-à-vis* questionnaire survey, face-to-face interviews, telephone interviews, degree of structure attached to question formats, resources and timescale constraints.

How were survey questions generated?

The manner in which survey questions are generated is an important issue because questions that are deemed relevant by researchers may not necessarily address the research question, never mind the concerns of the target population. Reports should show how the question items used in a survey were derived. Ideally, construction of question items in new questionnaires should involve some degree of participation from members of the target population through focus groups and pilot interviews.

Already validated survey questions, from previous studies, should be referenced.

Were survey questions validated?

New survey instruments, such as questionnaires, may need to undergo a process of validation before their application in a survey. Established instruments may also need to be revalidated if they were to be applied to a new kind of population. Validation is required to demonstrate that the instrument would measure exactly what it is designed to measure when applied to the target population in question.

For example, subjects may not understand the jargon contained in question items, for example 'insomnia'. Similarly, seemingly straightforward question items may be interpreted differently by subjects, for example *'How many hours a week do you spend on social activities?'* Here, the meaning of the term 'social activities' is unclear. It may or may not include things such as voluntary work, shopping, etc.

Was the survey instrument piloted?

Every survey instrument should ideally be piloted on a small population sample before commencement of the survey. This inescapable procedure is performed so as to iron out any potential or unforeseen problems that may affect the performance of that instrument. Any remarkable events that occur during this process should be addressed and stated in the survey report.

In addition, efforts made to counteract the effects of responder bias during validation should be included in the survey report.

Are details of survey instrument provided?

Details of the survey instrument should ideally be provided in the reporting of a survey. If a newly developed instrument is used, a copy of this should be included in the report.

Is the sampling frame justified?

The sampling frame in a cross-sectional survey can be described as the pool from which subjects are to be selected by random sampling. Sampling frames should, of course, be relevant to the target population and should be carefully chosen so as to avoid excluding large subgroups of that population, a potent source of sampling error (Table 4.2).

Table 4.2 Examples of sampling frames

Intended target population	Appropriate sampling frame
General population	Electoral register, valuation lists, postcode address file
Mother and baby	Register of births
Service users	Service provider registers
Doctors	Medical register

Beware of invitational sampling frames. An invitational sampling frame is said to occur wherever researchers appeal for people to participate in a survey, even if such respondents are then subjected to random sampling before selection. It is felt that people who volunteer themselves for participation are essentially different from those who do not, for example higher levels of motivation, anger, etc. (See volunteer bias.)

EXAMPLE

In the light of imminent elections, a poll (*cross-sectional survey*) is carried out on 5000 potential voters. In this poll, all potential voters in a town were invited to call a free phone number to register their voting intentions. In fairness to the pollsters, the voting intentions of every fifth caller only were noted. The results of this poll showed that political group X, a minority fringe organization, would win the elections by a 99% landslide, clearly a ridiculous prediction.

On reflection, pollsters attributed this anomaly to sampling error and concluded that the responders to their invitational sampling frame were much more motivated than was the average potential voter. A repeat poll of 5000 people conducted a week later avoided this error by randomly selecting potential voters from the town's electoral register, a methodologically superior sampling frame.

Was the chosen sampling design justified?

Ideally, survey participants should be randomly selected from a sampling frame, that is, 'random sampling'. All individuals in the sampling frame therefore have an equal probability of being selected for participation in the survey. Apart from simple random sampling, other frequently used sample designs include stratified random sampling, systematic random sampling, multistage random sampling, cluster sampling, quota sampling, etc. Details and justification for chosen methods should be stated in the survey report.

How was sample size determined?

It is most important that researchers should consult with a statistician regarding the sample size calculation of a survey. Inadequate sample size leads to the collection of unrepresentative information called 'sampling error'.

As a general rule, the greater the number of properties being measured in a survey (age, gender, ethnicity, socio-economic status, etc.) the larger the sample size needed in that survey. Furthermore, the estimated prevalence of measured properties also affects the sample size of a survey, as does the variability of that property in the general population. (See sample size calculations.)

What was response rate?

The response rate of a cross-sectional survey is of crucial importance. This is more the case with self-completed postal questionnaires than with face-to-face interviews or a survey of records. It is felt that those who do not respond to a questionnaire may have important characteristics that make them systematically different from those who do respond. Although there are no firm and fast rules on response rates, a response rate of 60–80% is what every cross-sectional survey should aspire to.

Low response rates can cause sampling error, that is, the gathering of unrepresentative information. If known, the profile of non-responders should be included in a survey report in order that the reader knows about their characteristics, such as age, ethnicity, socio-economic status, geographical location, etc. Non-response rate figures should include all cases of refusal, deaths or infirmity, subjects deemed ineligible during the selection process as well as partial responders. (Note: surveys of healthcare workers have notoriously low response rates!)

Were efforts made to ensure better response?

Efforts made in a cross-sectional survey to encourage better response rates should be included in survey reports. These may include the addition of an introductory covering letter or the use of a personalized introduction, such as *'Dear library member'* or *'Dear customer'*, etc.

Other methods include the sending of several postal reminders, telephone reminders, face-to-face reminders or even the offer of some sort of enticement. More ways of improving response rates include a guarantee of anonymity, the inclusion of a stamped self-addressed envelope or even the use of alternative access such as whilst sitting in hospital waiting rooms.

What do the results show?

Cross-sectional survey reports are mainly descriptive in nature. With descriptive survey reports, results are simply presented exactly as observed in the survey. Population measures, such as incidence rates or prevalence rates, or other more specific rates and percentages are commonly used measures when reporting the results of a survey. Descriptive survey reports can also feature comments on any trends or patterns identified in the survey along with differences between relevant subgroups of the population surveyed.

Survey reports can also be analytical in nature. With analytic reports, researchers go a step further than simply describing the result findings from a survey. Here, gathered data can be further explored with respect to a number of co-variables deemed relevant by the researchers. Such variables may include age groups, gender, disease severity, educational status, income, etc.

Such analytical exploration of the data from a survey is performed in order to make better sense of initial result observations and also in order to test any postulated hypotheses or relationships. Naturally, appropriate statistical tests are applied during this analytical process so as to generate accompanying *p*-values and confidence intervals.

Definitions of various population measures such as incidence and prevalence rates are included in the 'glossary of terms' at the end of the book.

Understanding mortality measures

Population mortality measures include the 'crude mortality rates', the 'specific mortality rates', the 'standardized mortality rates' and the 'standardized mortality ratio'. The meanings of the various mortality measures and how they are derived are described below.

Crude mortality rate

The crude mortality rate (CMR) provides information on the proportion of a defined population that die over a given period. The CMR is a crucial epidemiological measure as it allows us to monitor any changing death patterns in a population from one time period to another.

$$\text{CMR} = \frac{\text{deaths occurring over a given period}}{\text{number in population at midpoint of period} \times \text{length of period}} \times 1000$$

THE POPULATION

The population is usually defined by political (e.g. England and Wales population) or epidemiological (e.g. adult male diabetic population) imperatives.

THE TIME PERIOD

The time period is usually a calendar year but may be longer if the number of deaths in one calendar year is too small a figure.

TOTAL NUMBER OF PEOPLE IN POPULATION

An estimate for this figure can be obtained from the databases of the relevant census authorities in that population. The estimate is usually made for the midpoint of the said time period.

NUMBER OF DEATHS DURING THE SAID PERIOD

This figure can be obtained from the deaths register of that population.

CONSTANT

Fraction formed by the number of deaths and the total number in population is usually multiplied by 1000 or 100,000 in order to transform the otherwise highly decimalized figures to more readable figures. For example, $0.0000689 \times 100{,}000 = 6.89$ per 100,000 (population).

The main drawback of the CMR as a population measure, however, lies in the fact that it is directly derived from data on raw deaths in a population (i.e. a crude rate) and makes no allowances for certain structural population factors that can readily influence the observed death rates in any population.

Structural factors known to affect observed death rates in populations can include population sizes, gender distributions, age distributions, etc. However, the most crucial factor when making mortality rate comparisons between different populations is the age distributions of the different compared populations. As a general rule, the greater the proportion of aged people in a population, the higher would be the observed death rates in that population, that is, a pure age-related effect.

Specific mortality rate

Since different populations have different age or gender or socioeconomic structures, etc., which can in turn directly influence the data on observed death rates, the number of deaths in a population needs to be regarded in the context of the type of population in which they occurred.

For instance, in order to correct for the effects of different age structures in compared populations, the 'age-specific mortality rates' (ASMR) can be calculated instead of the crude mortality rates.

(Note: Age is used as an example of a structural population factor throughout this section even though other factors such as gender or social class are equally applicable.)

EXAMPLE

Consider the following mortality rate comparisons between populations A and B. Town A exists in a Third World country, whereas Town B exists in a developed European country. According to crude mortality rates, population A would appear to have better overall health than population B, as reflected by a lower crude mortality rate. This is despite the fact that population B probably has better healthcare facilities as would be expected in a developed country.

	Number of deaths in one year	Mid-year population		CMR per 1000 per year
Population A	986	86,935	(986/86,935) × 1000	11.34
Population B	657	45,563	(657/45,563) × 1000	14.42

When ASMRs are calculated for each age group, as shown below, it becomes clear that the higher crude mortality rate seen with population B is due to having a higher proportion of aged people. Hence, the effects of different age structures in populations A and B have been eliminated.

Age groups (years)	ASMR per 1000 per year		Per cent of population in age group	
	A	B	A	B
0–4	19.1	2.6	9.83	7.62
5–14	2.5	0.4	14.87	12.93
15–24	2.7	0.7	15.43	11.12
25–34	6.6	0.8	20.65	7.29
35–44	9.1	1.9	12.96	18.94
45–54	12.3	5.9	13.14	14.17
55–64	31.4	17.3	8.67	13.66
65–74	69.3	46.2	3.46	8.34
75–84	148.6	103.9	0.90	4.26
85+	291.7	216.6	0.09	1.67

However, it would be very inconvenient if ASMRs had to be calculated every time mortality comparisons are made in epidemiological studies, particularly since such comparisons can often be made between scores of different populations at a time.

This potential inconvenience is avoided in epidemiology by a process of standardization, which involves the use of 'standard' populations as benchmarks against which other populations can then be compared. Examples of such standard populations include the world population, European population, national population, regional population and so on.

Standardization can be performed in either of two ways.

DIRECT STANDARDIZATION METHODS

These involve use of the age distribution of the standard population. Here, the ASMRs from the study populations being compared are multiplied by the corresponding age-group proportions seen with the standard population to create standardized ASMRs. From the illustration below, the standardized ASMRs from populations A and B can be seen to be 25.09 and 14.69, respectively.

Age groups (years)	Age-group proportions in standard population	ASMR-A	Standardized ASMR-A	ASMR-B	Standardized ASMR-B
0–4	0.04	19.1	0.76	2.6	0.10
5–14	0.11	2.5	0.28	0.4	0.04
15–24	0.18	2.7	0.49	0.7	0.13
25–34	0.16	6.6	1.06	0.8	0.13
35–44	0.16	9.1	1.46	1.9	0.30
45–54	0.11	12.3	1.35	5.9	0.65
55–64	0.12	31.4	3.77	17.3	2.08
65–74	0.06	69.3	4.16	46.2	2.77
75–84	0.04	148.6	5.94	103.9	4.16
85+	0.02	291.7	5.83	216.6	4.33
Total	1.00		25.09		14.69

INDIRECT STANDARDIZATION METHODS

These involve use of ASMRs from the standard population. These rates can then be applied to any study population to determine the number of deaths that would be *expected* in that population in light of the numbers in each age group of that population. Comparing the observed number of deaths (O) with the expected number of deaths (E) creates a measure called a 'standardized mortality ratio' (SMR).

Age groups (years)	ASMR per 1000 per year in standard population	Age group total of population A	Expected number of deaths (E) $\frac{(1.86 \times 8546)}{1000}$	Observed number of deaths (O)	Standardized mortality ratio (SMR) (O/E) × 100
0–4	1.86	8546	16	164	1025

Age groups (years)	ASMR per 1000 per year in standard population	Age group total of population B	Expected number of deaths (E) $\frac{(1.86 \times 3472)}{1000}$	Observed number of deaths (O)	Standardized mortality ratio (SMR) (O/E) × 100
0–4	1.86	3472	7	9	129

An SMR equal to 100 means both the population under examination and the standard population have the same mortality picture. An SMR greater than 100 means the population under examination has a worse mortality picture than the standard population. An SMR less than 100 means the population under examination has a better mortality picture than the standard population.

Remember that standardization may be applied to other population parameters, such as gender, social class, etc.

P-value of SMR

A *p*-value can be worked out for an SMR by use of the chi-square statistic:

$$\chi^2 = \frac{(O - E)^2}{E}$$

Using population 'A' as an example:

$$\chi^2 = \frac{(164 - 16)^2}{16} = 1369$$

Looking along the $df = 1$ row on the chi-square distribution (Table iii, p. 57) $\chi^2 = 1369$ corresponds to $p < 0.001$. The SMR of 1025 quoted for population A is therefore strongly significant.

The *p*-value answers the question: 'What is the probability of obtaining an SMR value at least as different from 100 as observed, if no difference really existed between the mortality experience in both population A and the standard population?'

95% confidence interval of SMR

Standard error of SMR of population A:

$$= \frac{\sqrt{O}}{E} \times 100 = \frac{\sqrt{1025}}{16} \times 100 = 200$$

95% CI of population A SMR:

$$= 1025 \pm 1.96\ (200)$$
$$= 633 \text{ to } 1417$$

How do the results affect the care of my patients?

This aspect is concerned with how applicable the results of a survey are to the care of patients and how results may (if at all), change clinical practice.

- Survey results may have implications for your practice if the area of healthcare examined by the survey is directly relevant the patients in your care.
- Ensure that the subjects who participated in the survey are not essentially different from your patients in general.
- The results from a survey may have urgent implications for screening procedures in cases where detection has an impact on morbidity or mortality.
- The results of a survey may have implications for care provision where existing arrangements have been shown as not meeting the needs of service users.
- The results of a survey may be of limited use if changes are not likely to alter the course of the disease condition in question.
- The impact of survey results may be limited by resource issues in some clinical situations.

Again, this is where your clinical judgement based on experience and expertise comes into play.

Critical appraisal of prospective studies

5

Introduction

A prospective experiment is one that is conducted forwards in time. In a prospective cohort study, subjects are classified into groups depending on whether or not they are exposed to a risk factor. These groups of subjects, called 'cohorts' (Roman term meaning a tenth of a legion), are then followed over a time period after which exposed and non-exposed subjects are compared with regard to rates of development of an outcome of interest (Figure 5.1). This comparison between exposed and non-exposed groups is in order to identify any possible relationships that may exist between a risk factor and an outcome.

Prospective cohort studies

Prospective cohort studies can also provide valuable information about the strength of any observed relationship between risk factor and disorder. Other valuable insights that can be derived from a prospective study include:

- Information on any possible 'multiple effects' of a single risk factor.
- Evidence of a dose–effect relationship between risk factor and outcome.

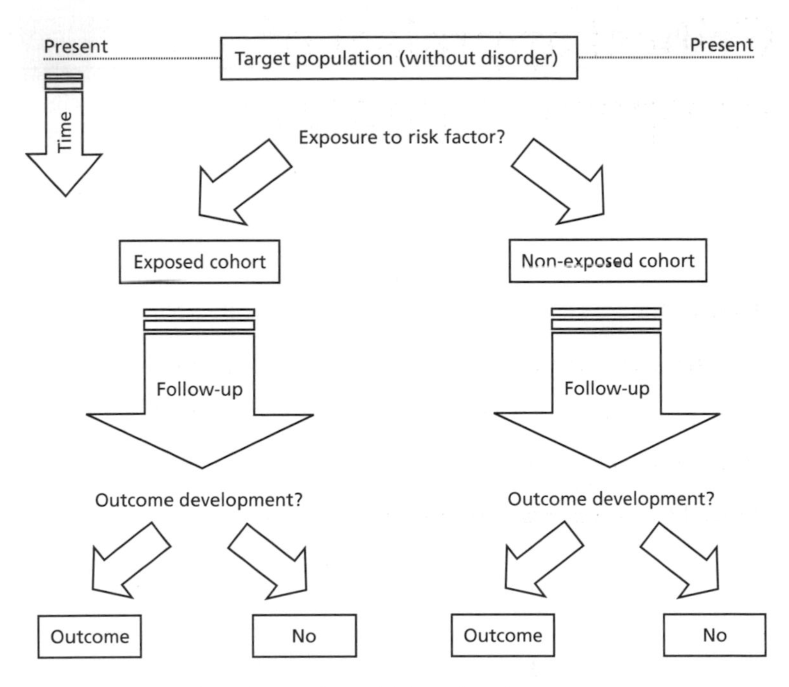

Figure 5.1 Prospective cohort study methdology flowchart.

- Data on the 'temporal relationship' that may exist between risk factor and outcome.
- Valuable 'prognostic information' provided by ongoing observations of other factors (apart from risk factor) that may affect outcome.
- Accurate information on disease 'incidence'. This is particularly the case with large studies.

Since cohorts are followed up in time, all relevant events that happen to each subject in a prospective study can be observed and noted as they occur. This reduces the potential for recall bias. Also much-reduced in prospective studies is the potential for confusion about causality between exposure and outcome, that is, which came first. This is because the exposure status of all subjects is known at the start of a prospective study before anyone develops the outcome of interest.

The drawbacks of prospective cohort studies are that they are expensive and time-consuming to conduct. They also need much follow up over prolonged periods, which can be difficult for both researchers and subjects alike. These disadvantages are even more pronounced with large-sized prospective cohort studies.

Example

In a prospective cohort study examining a possible link between cigarette smoking and ischaemic heart disease, two groups of subjects, 10,000 smokers and 10,000 non-smokers, were followed up over a 30-year period.

Apart from a ten-fold increase in the rates of ischaemic heart disease observed in the smokers group, results also showed that the median survival time, that is, the time from commencement of smoking to the development of ischaemic heart disease was 20 years (*temporal relationship*).

Further result analysis showed that a subset of experimental subjects who were smokers at the start of the study but who stopped smoking up to seven years after commencement had significantly lower rates of ischaemic heart disease compared to those who carried on smoking (*prognostic information*).

In addition to ischaemic heart disease, rates of other disorders, such as cerebrovascular disease, impotence, laryngeal cancer, chronic airway disease and lung cancer, were all significantly higher in the smokers group (*multiple effects of a single risk factor*).

The number of cigarettes smoked daily and the number of years of smoking showed a linear correlation to the risk of developing ischaemic heart disease (*dose–effect relationship*).

So, the critical appraisal of a prospective cohort study asks:

- Is the study design methodologically sound?
- What do the results show?
- How do the results affect the care of my patients?

Is the study design methodologically sound?

The issues discussed below are the main considerations when assessing the strengths and weaknesses of prospective cohort study design.

Are the exposure criteria described?

The criteria by which subjects were assessed as being exposed or non-exposed to a risk factor need to be clearly defined by researchers. These criteria should ideally be set out before the selection process. A lack of clarity on this issue can result in the erroneous acceptance into a study of control subjects who are exposed to the risk factor or of experimental subjects who have not been exposed to the risk factor, thereby raising fundamental questions about the validity of the study.

Wherever relevant, different grades of exposure to the risk factor should be recorded. This enables researchers to examine possible dose–effect relationships between risk factor and outcome later during the stage of result analysis.

Was the possibility of changing risk status addressed?

In prospective cohort studies, particularly in studies involving large sample sizes or prolonged follow-up durations, control subjects assessed as being unexposed at the start of the study may become exposed to the putative risk factor later on during the study. Similarly, experimental subjects confirmed as being exposed to a risk factor at the start of the study might cease to be exposed later on.

Measures to identify and address this changing risk status should be discussed in the report of a prospective cohort study. This is particularly relevant in prospective cohort studies where the cessation of exposure is not associated with a continued risk of outcome.

How was exposure measured?

The methods and instruments used in measuring exposure to risk factor in a prospective cohort study should be clearly described. Although some exposures can be measured in a straightforward way (e.g. first trimester lithium treatment or not?), others may require more sophisticated instruments (e.g. an eating-attitudes questionnaire or a body-image interview schedule). Exposure to a putative risk factor should be measured in the same way in both the exposed and unexposed groups of a prospective cohort study using validated instruments and methods wherever possible.

How were experimental subjects selected?

The mode of selection of participants into a study should be clearly stated and justified. Experimental subjects judged as being exposed to a risk factor should be as representative of the concerned target population as possible. A poorly representative sample weakens the validity of any inferences that can be made to that target population from the study results.

How were the control subjects selected?

The sampling frame from which control subjects were selected should also be clearly stated and justified. The general population is a sampling frame from which control subjects are commonly selected. However, in prospective cohort studies where occupational risk factors are being examined, 'healthy-worker' bias can be introduced if a general population control group is used. This bias results from the fact that members of the general population when compared to members of a specific occupational group are generally less healthy, worse educated, less aware, poorer, etc.

An important characteristic of the control subjects in a prospective cohort study is that they should *not* have been exposed to the putative risk factor and yet be similar to the exposed subjects in all other respects related to the likelihood of disease (such as age). Therefore, researchers should show how control cohorts were confirmed as meeting the non-exposure criteria of that study. Generally, the best practice when setting up a control group is to select unexposed subjects from a similar demographic, occupational or geographic setting as the exposed cohort.

How were outcomes measured?

The methods and instruments used in the measurement of outcomes in a prospective cohort study should be adequately described in the study report. Outcomes should ideally be measured in a similar way in both cohorts. Although some outcome events are easily demonstrable (e.g. death), other outcomes can only be demonstrated by more complicated means (e.g. self-esteem changes). Again, validated instruments and methods should be used in the measurement of outcomes in a study.

Is (are) the chosen outcome measure(s) justified?

Authors should justify their choice of outcome measure in a prospective cohort study. The chosen outcome measures should be reliable and validated as being truly reflective of the clinical outcome of interest. Outcome measures can include anything from directly measurable physical signs to serological or radiological events, psychological questionnaire scores, etc. (See surrogate endpoints, p. 128.)

Often, particularly with studies involving complex clinical outcomes, several outcome measures may need to be examined simultaneously. However, a Type I error becomes more likely with such multiple outcome measures because of the increased risk that one of those measures would show a significant observation by chance. Therefore, whenever multiple measures are being examined, the principal outcome measure of interest in that study should be stated.

Were relevant prognostic data collected?

When planning a prospective cohort study, other factors that may have important prognostic effects on the outcome should also be considered and identified. Data on these prognostic factors should be obtained from both the exposed and unexposed groups so that any significant differences can be taken into consideration when analysing results.

EXAMPLE

In the smoking and lung cancer prospective study described above, data should ideally be collected from the both groups of subjects regarding family histories of lung cancer, specific occupational hazards, low-tar or high-filter cigarettes, etc. Both groups of subjects can then be compared regarding any significant differences in these prognostic factors, differences that are then incorporated into the analysis of results.

Were the compared groups similar?

The compared groups in a study must be broadly similar at the start of the study with regards to parameters such as number of subjects in each group, gender distribution, age distribution, social class, etc. This is in order to ensure an even distribution of important confounding factors.

Was follow-up duration adequate?

Adequate follow-up duration, long enough to find a difference (if one existed) between the compared groups is usually determined based on clinical grounds. An unnecessarily prolonged follow-up duration would be a waste of resources, whereas an inadequate follow-up duration can introduce bias in a study. The usual practice is that the follow-up duration in a prospective cohort study should be reasonably longer than the duration in which outcome events are expected to occur.

Do the numbers add-up?

Prospective cohort studies, in particular those with large sample sizes or prolonged follow-up duration are prone to high drop-out rates.

Measures put in place to counteract attrition and actual drop-out rates should be stated. Also, a description of subjects who dropped out of a study should be given so that any systematic differences between these and those completing the study can be examined. This guards against errors that can occur when estimating the strength of relationship between risk factor and outcome.

How was sample size determined?

A sample size calculation should be performed prior to starting a prospective cohort study in order to reduce the chance of a Type II error. The size of a prospective cohort study is chiefly determined by the prevalence of disorder in question and the magnitude of risk posed by being exposed to the putative causal factor. In other words, larger-sized prospective cohort studies are necessary when examining rare diseases, or when examining exposures associated with small risk of disorder.

Were the appropriate statistical tests used?

Ensure that the appropriate statistical tests have been used in the analysis of the various types of data presented in the study results (*categorical/continuous, normal/skewed*, etc). (see Table 1.2, p. 5.)

What do the results show?

In appraising the results of a prospective cohort study it is advisable to make a quick-scan judgement as to whether the reported association between the variable factor and outcome is a beneficial or harmful one. This allows for a more logical approach when the assessing the results.

Harmful relationships

The relationship between variable(s) and outcome may be a harmful one.

EXAMPLE

A prospective cohort study examines a possible relationship between prematurity (*predictor variable*) and specific reading disorder (SRD) (*outcome*). One thousand premature babies and 1000 full-term babies all born within a one-year period were randomly selected from hospital registers. They were followed up from birth until school leaving age at 16 years. Assuming no drop-outs consider the following results.

No children	SRD (outcome)	No SRD	Total
Cohort (Prem)	600	400	1000
Control	200	800	1000
Total	800	1200	2000

Probability of outcome (risk) in exposed subjects
(p1) = 600/1000 = 0.6
Probability of outcome (risk) in control subjects
(p2) = 200/1000 = 0.2

RELATIVE RISK (p1/p2)

This is a ratio comparing the probability of an outcome in those exposed with the probability of that outcome in those unexposed:

$$\text{Relative risk (RR)} = 0.6/0.2 = 3$$

This means premature babies are three times more likely than full-term babies to develop specific reading disorder (SRD) according to this study.

$RR < 1$ Decreased risk
$RR = 1$ No difference in risk
$RR > 1$ Increased risk

ABSOLUTE RISK INCREASE (ARI) (p1 − p2)

This describes the difference in risk between both groups. It expresses the additional risk of an outcome following exposure to a risk factor.

$$= 0.6 - 0.2 = 0.4$$

Absolute risk increase (ARI) is similar to absolute risk reduction (ARR) (see below). Here, however, ARI is used because $p1 > p2$, that is, a harmful effect.

RELATIVE RISK INCREASE (RRI) (p1 − p2)/p2

This measure is a ratio. Here, the risk difference described above (i.e. the difference in the risk of developing an outcome between those exposed and those unexposed) is expressed as a proportion of the risk in those unexposed.

RRI = (p1 − p2)/p2
Risk of specific reading disorder (SRD) in premature babies (p1) = 0.6
Risk of SRD in control group (p2) = 0.2
Difference in risk (attributable risk) (p1 − p2) = 0.6 − 0.2 = 0.4
Relative risk increase (RRI) (p1 − p2)/p2 = 0.4/0.2 = 2

This means prematurity increases the risk of SRD by 200% according to this study.

Beneficial relationships

Conversely, the relationship between variable(s) and outcome may be beneficial.

EXAMPLE

A prospective cohort study examines the possible effect of prolonged breastfeeding (*variable*) on measles infection in young children (*outcome*). In this study, two adjacent rural communities with contrasting breastfeeding practices were examined. The practice of prolonged breastfeeding (more than two years) found in one community was seen as taboo in the other community where women never breastfed for more than six months after birth. Over a ten-year period, trained health visitors who confirmed all events of measles infection followed up all children born in these two distinct communities until their fifth birthday. Assuming no immunization programme and zero mortality and drop-out rates, consider the following results.

No infants	Measles	No measles	Total
Two-year breastfed	20	80	100
Six-month breastfed	40	60	100
Total	60	140	200

Probability of outcome in exposed subjects (p1) = 20/100 = 0.2
Probability of outcome in control subjects (p2) = 40/100 = 0.4

RELATIVE RISK (p1/p2)

The ratio comparing the probability of outcome in those exposed (to prolonged breastfeeding) with the probability of outcome in those unexposed.

Relative risk (RR) = 0.2/0.4 = 0.5

According to this study, therefore, children breastfed for at least two years are half as likely (twice as unlikely) to develop measles infection when compared with children breastfed for up to six months (reciprocal of 0.5 = 2.0).

ABSOLUTE RISK REDUCTION (ARR) (ABSOLUTE BENEFIT INCREASE) (ABI)

Absolute risk reduction (ARR) simply describes the risk difference or reduction in risk of an outcome following exposure to a variable factor.

$$\begin{aligned} \text{ARR} &= \text{p2} - \text{p1} \\ &= 0.4 - 0.2 \\ &= 0.2 \end{aligned}$$

ARR is similar to ARI (see above). Here, however, ARR is used because p2 > p1, that is, a beneficial effect.

RELATIVE RISK REDUCTION (RRR) (p2 − p1)/p2

Also called 'relative benefit increase' (RBI), RRR is a similar concept to RRI. Here, the risk difference, that is, the difference in the risk of developing outcome (*measles infection*) between those exposed to variable (*prolonged breastfeeding*) and those unexposed is expressed as a proportion of the risk of those unexposed.

Risk of measles in exposed group (p1) = 0.2
Risk of measles in control group (p2) = 0.4
Difference in risk = 0.4 − 0.2 = 0.2
Relative risk reduction = 0.2/0.4 = 0.5 (50%)

This means prolonged breastfeeding decreases risk of measles by 50% according to this study. In other words, half the 'control' children who developed measles would not have done so, had they had prolonged breastfeeding.

Absolute versus relative measures

RRR and RRI are ratios and thus are able to convey a sense of proportional reduction or increase in risk. They are, therefore, easier to relate to than absolute measures, such as ARR or ARI. However, the main disadvantage of RRR and RRI is that, as ratios, they are unable to discriminate between huge and negligible absolute effects. Absolute measures like ARR or ARI have this capacity.

The advantages and disadvantages of relative and absolute measures are illustrated in the example below which has been borrowed from the number-needed-to-treat (NNT) discussion in the clinical trials section.

EXAMPLE

Two vaccines, A and B, having been tested, respectively, on two similarly sized populations are reported as reducing the risk of influenza (*outcome*) in the elderly. According to the results tabulated below, when compared with placebo, both vaccines reduced the influenza rates recorded in their respective populations by 50%, that is, the same RRR value of 0.5.

Vaccine A	No influenza	Influenza	Total
Vaccinated	600,000	400,000	1,000,000
Control	200,000	800,000	1,000,000
Total	800,000	1,200,000	2,000,000

A: $\frac{0.8 - 0.4}{0.8}$ RRR same as B: $\frac{0.00008 - 0.00004}{0.00008}$

Vaccine B	No influenza	Influenza	Total
Vaccinated	999,960	40	1,000,000
Control	999,920	80	1,000,000
Total	1,999,880	120	2,000,000

Because of a large difference in the baseline population susceptibility (*prevalence*) to influenza, the numbers of influenza cases seen in the respective populations differ markedly. In a case such as this, an RRR measure can be misleading because it fails to convey the fact that vaccine A actually prevented Influenza at a rate of 400,000 cases per million elderly people who received it compared with a rate of 40 cases per million elderly people with vaccine B.

With the above scenarios the ARR for vaccines A and B would be:

ARR = p2 − p1
Vaccine A: 0.8 − 0.4 = 0.4 (40%)
Vaccine B: 0.00008 − 0.00004 = 0.00004 (0.004%)

What a difference! By retaining 'p2' in its formula, ARR takes into account the underlying baseline population susceptibility to influenza and, therefore, reflects the raw absolute treatment effects. Unfortunately, since ARR and ARI are absolute measures and not ratios, they cannot convey the easily digestible proportional reductions or increases in risk, which drug salespeople love to quote.

(Note: Number-needed-to-treat (NNT), number-needed-to-harm (NNH) and 'risk/benefit' analysis are discussed in the randomized clinical trials section.)

How do the results affect the care of my patients?

This aspect is concerned with how applicable the results of a prospective cohort study are to the care of patients and how they may (if at all) change your practice.

Even when a prospective cohort study fulfils all the validity criteria and has demonstrated a beneficial or harmful relationship between tested variables, questions still have to be asked by clinicians, such as:

- There may be implications for your practice if the area of healthcare examined by a prospective cohort study is directly relevant to the patients in your care.
- Ensure that the subjects who participated in the prospective cohort study are not essentially different from your patients.
- The results of a prospective cohort study may have implications for health education with respect to your patients who may share the risk factor in question.
- Resource issues may limit the overall impact of a prospective cohort study particularly with respect to health education and dissemination of information.

As ever, this is where your clinical judgement based on experience and expertise comes into play.

Critical appraisal of retrospective studies

6

Introduction

Retrospective studies examine a research question by look backwards in time. In case-control studies – a type of retrospective study – subjects confirmed with a disease (*cases*) are compared with non-diseased subjects (*control subjects*) regarding past exposure to a putative risk factor (*variable*). Therefore, both groups are compared for possible past exposure to a risk factor (Figure 6.1).

Retrospective (case-control) studies

As was discussed earlier (Chapter 5), the ability and motivation to recall past exposure to a risk factor may vary in subjects depending on whether or not they have actually had a disorder. It is understandable, therefore, why retrospective studies are inextricably linked with some degree of recall bias. In fact, recall bias is the major drawback of retrospective studies.

Another potential source of bias that may occur in some retrospective studies is that of 'ascertaining causality'. Because of the retrospective

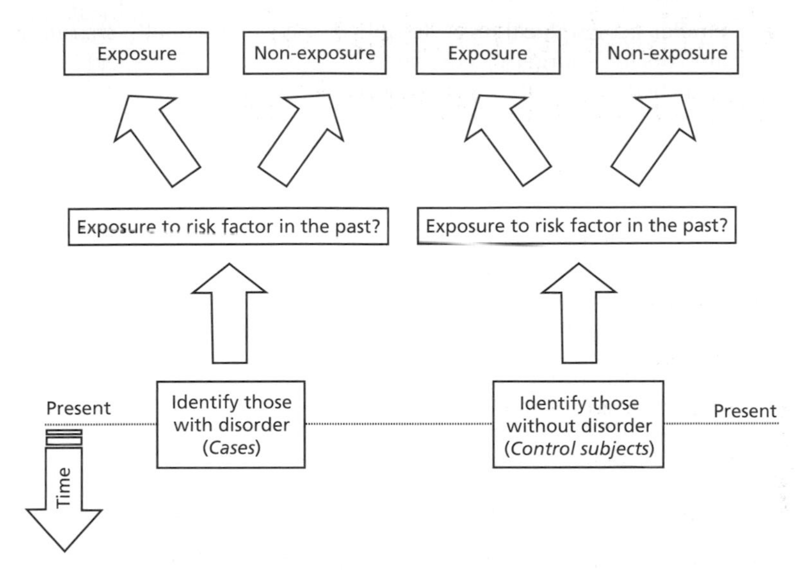

Figure 6.1 Case-control study methodology flowchart.

nature of the design, it may be difficult in some studies to determine which was the initial event in the case group subjects: exposure to a risk factor or the development of outcome.

However, the advantages of retrospective studies are many. They are relatively quick and inexpensive to set up. They are an efficient approach to research when the disorder in question has a prolonged course or when many hypotheses on causation are being tested.

Retrospective designs are particularly practical when the disease in question is a rarely occurring one or one with a long latent (*asymptomatic*) period. Imagine how many subjects would have to be recruited or how lengthy the follow-up duration would have to be if prospective designs were used to examine a rare disease, such as progeria, or a condition with a long latent period, such as Creutzfeld–Jacob disease.

Matched and unmatched case-control studies

The design of case-control studies may or may not involve a matching procedure. In unmatched case-control studies, a control population (*without disorder*) is simply selected based on other criteria, such as 'living in a similar geographical area', 'pupils of the same school', 'sharing a common doctor's surgery', 'customers of the same butcher's shop', etc.

In matched case-control studies, each unexposed control subject is chosen in such a way as to match a case subject on a finite set of criteria that are regarded as potential confounding factors. These criteria usually include age, gender, ethnicity, social class, etc. (see overmatching, p. 62). Matching renders the data collected from both groups easier to compare, it addresses any identified potential confounding factors and, to a less important extent, matching may allow for slightly smaller sample sizes than would be otherwise necessary with unmatched studies.

Thus, critical appraisal of a retrospective study asks:

- Is the study design methodologically sound?
- What do the results show?
- How do the results affect the care of my patients?

Is the study design methodologically sound?

The issues discussed below are the main considerations when assessing the strengths and weaknesses of a case-control study design.

How were the cases selected?

The source from which cases were obtained is an important issue in a case-control study. Subjects with disorder are readily available from large hospital or specialist settings (usually where researchers work) and often, in order to save time and resources, many studies recruit their case subjects mainly from these specialized populations.

However, recruitment of case subjects from specialist settings has a high potential for prevalence bias. This is because case subjects recruited from specialist settings can be systematically different from non specialist-setting sufferers of that same disorder. For example, subjects recruited from specialist settings may have more chronic or more severe disorders, they may be more motivated to seek help or may be more able to afford specialist care, etc.

Alternatively, case subjects can be recruited from the general population or from primary care settings. This usually yields a more representative sample, that is, containing sufferers with different grades and variants of that disorder. However, this method can be more expensive and time-consuming to carry out. Researchers should justify and describe their selection methods in detail.

How were the control subjects obtained?

Generally, control subjects (*matched* or *unmatched*) should ideally be selected from a similar source as the case subjects. This is because systematic differences can occur between groups that have been selected from different sources. Increasingly, people with a different type of disorder are being used as control subjects in retrospective case-control studies. The purpose of using 'ill control subjects' is to reduce the impact of recall bias on study results. Often a case-control study will have two (or more) sets of controls, such as one hospital-based and the other a population-based. This is often performed to increase the validity of eventual result findings.

Are the groups similar?

Subjects in the case groups and control groups in retrospective studies should be broadly similar in terms of parameters such as the number of subjects in each group, age distribution or other demographic characteristics. The main difference between the groups should be their disease status. In other words, the case group subjects already have the disorder, whereas the control group subjects do not.

Are there sufficient numbers?

The number of subjects involved in a retrospective study should be sufficiently large in order to reduce the chance of a Type II error. Large numbers also increase the validity and robustness of any conclusions that can be drawn from the results of a retrospective study (see sample size calculation, p. 18).

How was the disorder confirmed in the cases?

The disorder being investigated in a retrospective case-control study should be confirmed as being present in the case subjects and absent in the control subjects prior to recruitment into the study. These assessments should be carried out in a similar manner for both groups of subjects using validated and objective methods in order to reduce observer bias. The diagnostic criteria for 'caseness' used in a retrospective study should be stated.

Were there equal opportunities?

Control subjects in case-control studies should ideally be selected on the basis that they should have had similar opportunities for exposure to proposed variable factor as subjects in the case group. The example below illustrates this often-overlooked flaw in retrospective study designs.

EXAMPLE

A retrospective study examined the association between development of post-traumatic stress disorder (PTSD) and exposure to heavy military combat. One thousand 'suffering' Vietnam veterans were matched and compared with 1000 control veterans. A control sample, comprising 'syndrome-free' Vietnam veterans would be a methodologically better idea than a sample comprising 'syndrome-free' peace keeping veterans. This is because the latter group of veterans would have had less opportunity to be exposed to the proposed causative factor – heavy military combat.

Was exposure status in both groups measured similarly?

Exposures to risk factor should ideally be measured using similar methods in both groups. It would be methodologically, silly therefore, to measure exposure to heavy combat in the post-traumatic stress disorder (PTSD) group by studying service records whilst relying only on personal accounts with the control group. Ideally, assessors should be blind to the disease states in order to reduce observer bias where assessors unconsciously search for evidence of exposure with more vigour in case subjects than they do with control subjects.

Observer bias in case-control studies can be further reduced with the use of objective methods of measurement, such as structured interviews or actual records, as opposed to subjective methods, such as patient recall or collateral information.

Are there sufficient numbers?

The necessary sample size should be determined before the start of a retrospective study in order to reduce the chance of a Type II error (see sample size calculation, p. 18).

What do the results show?

Issues that are likely to be raised when appraising retrospective case-control studies are deliberately presented here as a clinical vignette.

Example

In a retrospective study examining possible links between occupational exposure to asbestos (*variable*) and lung cancer (*outcome*), 1000 proven lung cancer deaths spanning a 10-year period were randomly selected from several hospital case registers. The concerned cases were matched for age, gender and illness duration, with 1000 proven non-lung cancer deaths. Occupational histories and employment records of all 2000 subjects in the study were examined for significant (≥6 months) exposure to asbestos. The results are summarized below.

	Asbestos exposure	No exposure	Total
Lung cancer	60	940	1000
Control	2	998	1000

Odds

Probabilities may be easier to relate to than odds for most people. However, because retrospective studies look backwards in time, risk cannot be logically described in terms of probabilities. Instead, odds are used to approximate risk. The odds of an event are defined as the probability of an event occurring compared with the probability of that event not occurring.

$$\text{Odds} = \text{probability}/(1 - \text{probability})$$

The odds that lung cancer subjects were exposed to asbestos

$$\text{oE} = 60/940 = 0.064$$

The odds that control subjects were exposed to asbestos

$$\text{oC} = 2/998 = 0.002$$

Odds-ratio

Odds-ratios are similar in principle to the 'relative risk' concept commonly used in prospective studies. An odds-ratio is defined as the ratio of the odds of an event occurring in the experimental group (oE) compared with the odds of same event in the control group (oC).

$$\text{Odds ratio (OR)} = \text{oE}/\text{oC} = 0.064/0.002 = 32$$

This means that the odds of past asbestos exposure in patients with lung cancer are 30 times greater than the odds of same exposure in patients without lung cancer. It does *not* mean that asbestos exposure is 30 times more likely than normal to cause lung cancer, that is, not relative risk!

OR $<$ 1 suggests exposure reduces outcome
OR $=$ 1 suggests exposure has no effect
OR $>$ 1 suggests exposure increases outcome

Risk versus odds

Because of different denominators, an odds measure can only offer an approximate estimation of risk. Nevertheless, in addition to describing risk from a retrospective perspective, odds and odds ratios are also often used in prospective studies, randomized clinical trials and systematic reviews. This is because the odds measure also possesses certain mathematical advantages over straightforward risk values, advantages that allow for more flexibility during statistical analyses.

Moreover, when the risk of an event is low, the odds of that event are almost equal to the risk. In fact, with very low risk events, odds can be assumed to be equal to risk, as shown in Table 6.1.

Table 6.1 Relationship between risk and odds

Number of events per thousand	950	750	500	250	100	25	1	0.1
Risk of event (*event rate/total*)	0.95	0.75	0.5	0.25	0.10	0.025	0.001	0.0001
Odds of event (*event rate/ non-event rate*)	19	3	1	0.33	0.11	0.026	0.001	0.0001

Retrospective (cohort) studies

This term describes studies in which cohorts are followed up from a time point in the past (Figure 6.2). Here, recruitment into the study is of

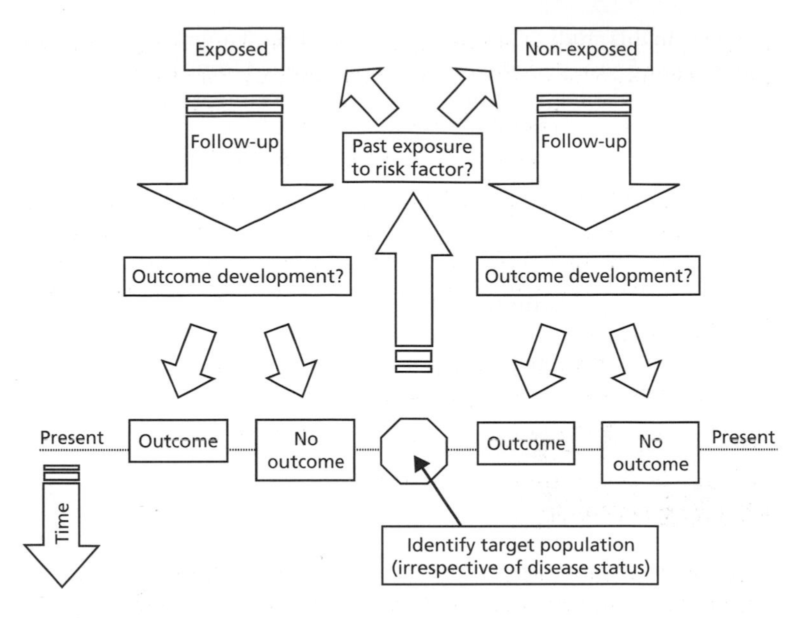

Figure 6.2 Restrospective cohort study methodology flow chart.

an unclassified sample of subjects chosen irrespective of their disease status. A history of exposure or non-exposure to a putative risk factor in the *past* is then determined in every subject.

Having ascertained exposure or non-exposure, all relevant events that have since occurred to the respective subjects are then explored and recorded. Both groups are finally compared regarding the presence of an outcome.

Therefore, the methodology of a retrospective cohort study is somewhat similar to that of a prospective cohort study in that the exposure to risk factor is determined initially and only then are cohorts followed up regarding any subsequent events, including the development of outcome. As with any retrospective study, however, the main drawback of retrospective cohort studies is the potential for subject recall bias when ascertaining past exposures to risk factor.

EXAMPLE OF A RETROSPECTIVE COHORT STUDY

A retrospective cohort study is designed to examine an alleged harmful relationship between a brand of silicon breast prosthesis (*risk factor*) and increasing reports of polyarthritis (*outcome*) in breast augmentation patients. In this study, 500 subjects who had breast augmentation procedures over a 5-year period were randomly selected from a plastic surgery database. Implantation of the Sellotec brand of breast prosthesis (*risk factor*) at the time of operation was then checked for in all subjects.

From surgical records, 166 subjects were confirmed as having received the Sellotec prosthesis (*exposed*), whereas 334 subjects were confirmed as not having received the Sellotec prosthesis (*unexposed*). Following this, standardized face-to-face interviews, hospital records, serological tests and standard physical examinations were used to test for evidence of polyarthritis, with assessors being blind to the exposure status of the subjects.

Assuming there were no deaths or untraceable cases, consider the following results.

	Polyarthritis	No polyarthritis	Total
Sellotec	33	133	166
Non-Sellotec	5	329	334
Total	38	462	500

Risk of polyarthritis in the Sellotec group (p1)

$$= 33/166 = 0.199$$

Risk of polyarthritis in the non-Sellotec group (p2)

$$= 5/334 = 0.015$$

Relative risk (RR) of polyarthritis with implantation of Sellotec prosthesis

$$= p1/p2 = 0.199/0.015 = 13.3$$

Therefore, breast augmentation with the Sellotec prosthesis is associated with a ten-fold risk of polyarthritis compared to non-Sellotec breast augmentation. Note that comparisons can only be made with the control group that has been used. Therefore, the relative risk of polyarthritis with Sellotec compared to the general population cannot be determined from this study because a general population control group was not used.

How do the results affect the care of my patients?

This step is concerned with how applicable the results of a retrospective study are to the care of patients and how they may (if at all) change your practice.

Even when a retrospective study fulfils the ideal methodological criteria and has been able to show an association between an outcome and exposure to a variable factor, questions still have to be asked by clinicians, such as:

- Retrospective study results may have implications for your practice if the area of healthcare examined is directly relevant the patients in your care.
- Ensure that the subjects who participated in the retrospective study are not essentially different from your patients.
- The results from a retrospective study may have urgent implications for health education and dissemination of information to those patients under your care who may be currently exposed to the risk factor in question.
- Resource limitations may limit the impact of retrospective study results particularly with respect to health education and dissemination of information.
- Are there useful insights to be drawn from such studies regarding better care for patients?

This is where your clinical judgement based on experience and expertise comes into play. (See randomized clinical trial section Chapter 7 for 'risk/benefit' analysis.)

Critical appraisal of randomized clinical trials

7

Introduction

In a randomized clinical trial, a defined human population with a defined problem is randomly allocated to two or more comparable treatment conditions for a defined period. Outcomes are then compared between the groups. Throughout this chapter, the term 'clinical trial' is used in referring to phase III clinical trials.

Randomized clinical trials

Randomized clinical trials (RCT) are the generally accepted gold standard of medical research. In conducting RCTs, researchers observe stringent methodological guidelines based on sound scientific reasoning. This safeguards the robustness and validity of the result findings. RCTs test hypotheses on the treatment of disease, unlike prospective and retrospective studies, which test hypotheses on disease aetiology or prognosis.

As with any kind of clinical study involving live subjects, obtaining approval from an ethics committee is a prerequisite for conducting an RCT.

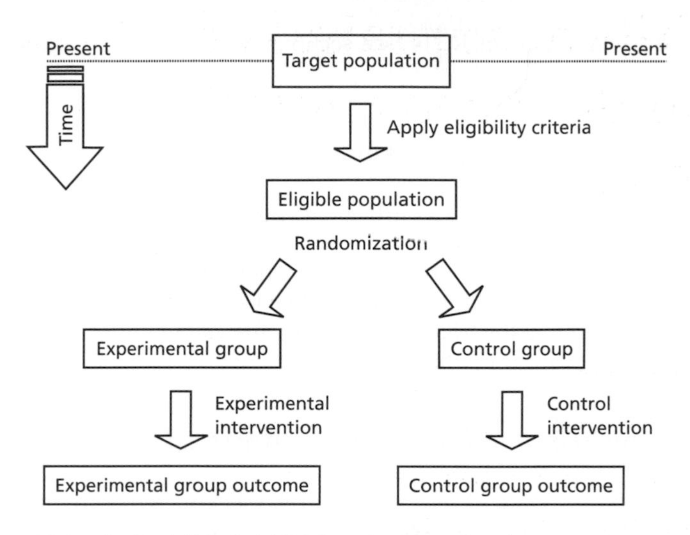

Figure 7.1 Randomized clinical trial (RCT) methodology flowchart.

Issues considered by ethics committees include the nature and purpose of intended study, study methodology, confidentiality issues, informed consent procedure, etc. This protective mechanism serves to protect patients from being subjected to poorly designed scientific experiments.

The critical appraisal of an RCT asks:

- Is the study design methodologically sound?
- What do the results show?
- How do the results affect the care of my patients?

Is the study design methodologically sound?

The issues discussed below are the main considerations when assessing the strengths and weaknesses of clinical trial design.

Was a sample size calculation performed?

A sample size calculation should be performed before the start of an RCT in order to ascertain the minimum number of subjects needed for the required power of that trial. Sample size calculations and the assumptions on which such calculations were based should be clearly stated in the report of RCTs (see sections on sample size calculations and open trials, p. 18).

How were the subjects selected?

The method of selection of participants into a trial needs to be clearly stated and justified. Selection methods that involve a random sampling of participants create the best representation of the target population because all eligible candidates would then have had an equal chance of being selected into the trial, strengthening the validity of any inferences drawn to the target population.

Were inclusion and exclusion criteria applied?

The inclusion and exclusion criteria observed in the selection process of a trial must be clearly stated. These criteria govern the eligibility for participation or disqualification from a trial. These criteria should be carefully set out, even before the commencement of a trial in order to minimize selection bias.

Wherever applicable, inclusion criteria should be based on recognized diagnostic criteria. Exclusion criteria that are too stringent may, however, introduce 'exclusion bias', as the study sample then becomes less representative of the target population.

Is the randomization procedure described?

The randomization procedure used in a trial should be clearly described in the trial report. Randomization, that is, the random allocation of study participants into the various groups of a trial can be done using any of several recognized methods including computer generated random numbers, randomization tables, etc. Randomization ensures that confounding factors within subjects that may affect the study outcome have an equal chance of being present in all the groups of a trial.

Were the compared groups similar?

Subjects in the various groups of a clinical trial should be similar at the start of the trial with regard to relevant parameters, such as number of subjects in each group, gender distribution, severity of illness, age distribution, etc. The purpose of this is to ensure an even distribution of confounding factors that may otherwise bias the results.

Was 'blinding' in effect?

The blinding procedure needs to be clearly stated in the trial report. Clinicians and subjects should both be blind to the nature of treatment the subjects are receiving. Blinding is important as it reduces bias in the way that subjects report their symptoms and the way clinicians observe beneficial or harmful effects thereby ensuring that the groups remain similar in all aspects (except treatment) after baseline.

The integrity of the blinding process can be examined during a trial by asking assessors and subjects questions as to which treatment group they think a subject should belong. Flaws in the blinding process are suspected if either subjects or assessors systematically 'get it right'.

Were the groups treated equally?

Apart from the experimental and control treatments, all other aspects of a trial must be of such nature that the groups within the trial receive equal and identical treatment. This minimizes the chance of performance bias and ensures that any differences in outcome can be ascribed to differences in experimental and control treatments alone. Groups that are treated equally in a trial is a desirable consequence of 'blinding'.

Were the treatment interventions clearly described?

The exact nature of the compared treatment interventions used in a randomized trial should be precisely defined. Control group interventions should be as clearly described as experimental group interventions. Descriptions of medicinal interventions should include exact dosages or range of dosages, along with the methods employed to ensure that the administrations of such interventions were standardized.

Ambiguity about treatment interventions raises doubts about the exact nature of the properties being compared and the treatment effects reported thereof. This ambiguity also insinuates that the treatments may not have been properly administered in the trial.

Were the chosen outcome measures appropriate?

The outcome measures observed in a trial should essentially reflect the outcome of interest, and the choice of outcome measure should be clearly justified by the authors. Outcome measures should be reliable and validated as being truly reflective of the outcome being measured.

Often, in order to examine several important aspects of a trial outcome, several outcome measures may be observed simultaneously. However, use of multiple outcome measures in a study can also increase the risk of Type I error. Hence, measures used in a trial to guard against this in a study should be stated, such as identifying one principal outcome measure that is given more importance than others.

Was there adequate follow-up?

The end-point of a randomized trial should be determined before the start of a trial and should be clearly stated in the trial report. The determination of a trial end-point, that is, the duration of follow-up that would be needed in order to find a difference in the compared groups is usually based on clinical reasoning. Some diseases and treatments, such as 'benefits of aspirin after myocardial infarction', may require a 5–10-year follow-up period, whereas 'influenza vaccination and 'flu prevention in the elderly' may need only a few months of follow-up.

Was an intention-to-treat analysis performed?

Data on all patients entering into a trial should be analysed with respect to the groups to which they were initially randomized, regardless of whether they received or completed the treatment to which they were allocated. Therefore, the data on a given trial subject who was allocated to Treatment A would have to be computed along with the data on all subjects who were similarly allocated to Treatment A, even if for some reason this particular subject ended up receiving Treatment B.

Note that in some kinds of trials (e.g. a trial simply interested in the physiological effects of a drug as opposed to the efficacy of that drug when used in practice), comparisons based on actual treatments received would be more appropriate than an intention-to-treat based comparison.

Do the numbers add up?

All subjects involved at the start should be clearly accounted for at the end of a trial. Accounting for all subjects who entered into a trial (including drop-outs) at the end prevents errors in estimating the overall treatment effects. The 'attrition' or drop-out rate is the proportion of patients who drop out for whatever reasons prior to the planned end-point of a trial. Reasons for attrition often include withdrawal from trial, deaths, migration, unexplained loss to follow-up, etc.

Data on drop-out subjects can be incorporated into the overall results in some pragmatic clinical trials. This can be done by any one of several methods, including the 'worst case scenario' method and the 'last data carried forward' method.

WORST CASE SCENARIO

When comparing the experimental and control groups in a trial, this method assumes a poor outcome for drop-outs from whichever group fared better and a good outcome for drop-outs from the group that fared worse. The idea therefore, is to be as conservative as possible when estimating how drop-outs from a group would have fared had they remained in the trial. In other words, assume a worst case scenario (Figure 7.2).

LAST DATA CARRIED FORWARD

Here, subjects who drop out of a trial for whatever reason should have their last recorded data before dropping out carried forward to the end of the trial. These 'brought-forward' data are then incorporated into the overall analysis of whichever group to which they originally belonged. Differences in drop-out rates and the timing of such drop-outs (early or late stages of a trial) influence the estimation of treatment effects, as explained below.

EXAMPLE

A 30-week trial compares a new anti-depressant drug with a control drug. One hundred similarly depressed subjects were recruited and randomized into experimental and control groups.

Twenty subjects (obviously still depressed) dropped out of the control group after one week and their 'still depressed' data were carried

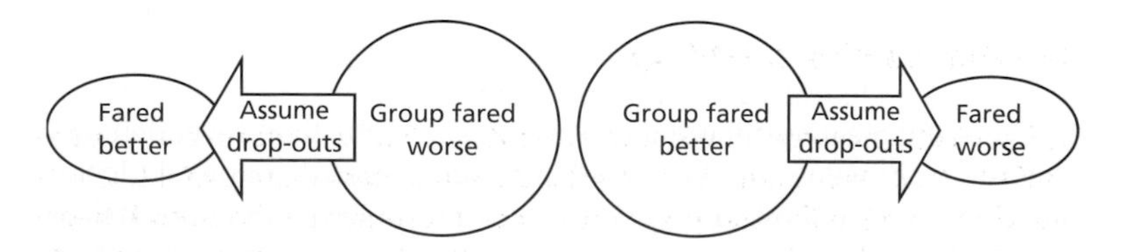

Figure 7.2 Worst case scenario.

forward for analysis at the end of the trial. The resulting effect would be a worsening of the overall control group results. By worsening the control group results, such drop-outs indirectly strengthen the magnitude of benefits obtained from treatment with the new drug.

This is a clinically important effect because the reasons for dropping out of a trial, such as adverse side-effects, non-compliance, morbidity, etc., are all clinically important issues, which should ideally be reflected in the overall result.

Conversely, if after one week, 20 subjects (obviously still depressed) dropped out of the treatment group, their 'still depressed' data would be carried forward for analysis at the end of the trial. The resulting effect would be a worsening of the overall treatment group results. By worsening the treatment group results, such drop-outs essentially cause a reduction in the magnitude of the treatment effects of the new drug.

Again, this is a clinically important effect because it gives the true picture regarding the overall clinical performance of the new drug.

Drop-outs that occur in the 29th week of the trial would have less impact on the overall results than drop-outs that occur in the first week. This is because week 29 data are likely to be very similar to the eventual completion data at week 30.

Were the statistical tests used appropriate?

The appropriate statistical tests should be applied in the analysis of the different types of data presented in a trial (*categorical/continuous, normal/skewed*, etc.). (See Table 1.2, p. 5.)

Miscellaneous clinical trial design issues

Surrogate end-points

A 'surrogate end-point' is an event that is regarded as being highly correlated, indicative or predictive of a clinically meaningful outcome in a trial. When used in clinical trials, surrogate end-points are substituted for the more clinically meaningful outcomes.

Clinically meaningful outcomes are those events that the patient and clinicians ultimately want to avoid, for example death, paralysis, loss of hearing, infertility, etc. Surrogate end-points, on the other hand, are biological markers, laboratory measures or physical signs that are used to replace clinically meaningful outcomes in a study.

Surrogate end-points are often used in studies where observance of the actual outcomes of interest would be highly impractical, invasive, costly or would involve too long a follow-up duration. Surrogate end-points can also help reduce the required sample size of a study when the actual outcome of interest is a rare event.

The main concern with the use of surrogate end-points is that of validity. Surrogate end-points should be already proven as being truly reflective or truly indicative of an outcome of interest, if they are to be used in a study. Use of unproven surrogate end-points can introduce 'information bias' where the properties being measured differ from the clinical outcome of interest in a study.

Furthermore, surrogate end-points may only reflect a limited aspect of a clinical outcome, or may simultaneously reflect another process besides that of the clinical outcome. In these instances, the suggestion would be that the actual disease process might be independent of the surrogate end-points being used. A poor dose–effect correlation with outcome of interest can also be a limitation when using some surrogate end-points. Results from studies that have used poorly derived or unproven surrogate end-points can be highly misleading. Table 7.1 highlights a few examples from the literature, where the observed surrogate end-point indicators of clinical improvement have not necessarily resulted in improvements of clinically meaningful outcomes.

Hawthorne effect

The Hawthorne effect refers to those clinical improvements that occur in study subjects just as a result of being participants in a trial. This

Table 7.1 Examples of surrogate end-points used in randomized clinical trials involving several disorders

Disorder under study	Clinically meaningful outcome	Surrogate end-point
Leukaemia	Mortality rate changes	Five-year survival rate changes
Schizophrenia	'Sanity'	Questionnaire score changes
Heart failure	Mortality rate changes	LV ejection fraction changes
HIV infection	Non-progression to AIDS	CD4 count changes
Osteoporosis	Fracture prevention rates	Bone density changes
Hypercholesterolaemia	Prevention of myocardial infarct	Serum cholesterol changes
Bowel cancer	Mortality rate changes	Tumour size changes

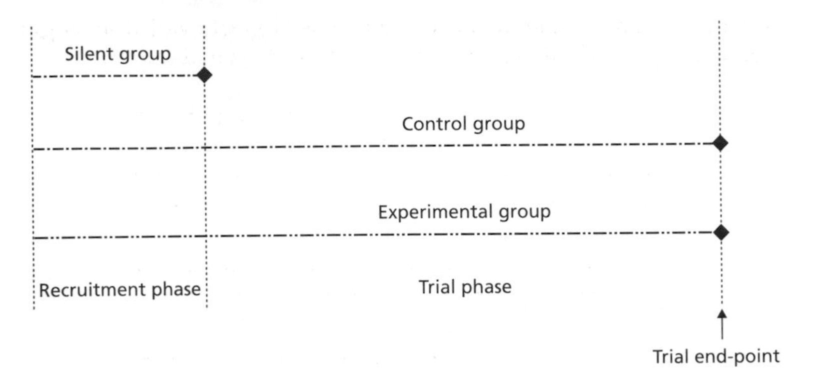

Figure 7.3 Counteracting the Hawthorne effect.

phenomenon occurs because mere clinical contact in a study alone can have a positive 'feel-good' effect on the way study subjects perceive their symptoms. Needless to say, this effect can produce artificially encouraging data on the beneficial effects experimental and control treatments.

To counteract the Hawthorne effect, a third 'silent' group may be created in addition to the experimental and control groups. This third group would usually have no further contact with the trial after the recruitment phase. Results of the silent and control groups can then be compared to assess for Hawthorne effect at the end of the trial (Figure 7.3).

Randomization

FIXED RANDOMIZATION METHODS

Simple randomization

These include the tossed coin, computer-generated random numbers and random number tables. These simple methods are best used with large samples where they are able to generate roughly equal numbers in the groups eventually. Their use in smaller sized studies usually leads to imbalance between groups or between subgroups.

Randomized permuted blocks

Here, the randomization of subjects to *all* the groups of a study is performed after every *n* number of sequential recruitments. This technique is useful for small-sized studies and studies of long duration where it can ensure that roughly comparable numbers of subjects are allocated to all study groups at any point in the process. Permuted blocks are used in a random order and can even be deliberately varied in length (Figure 7.4) to make it more difficult for researchers to decipher.

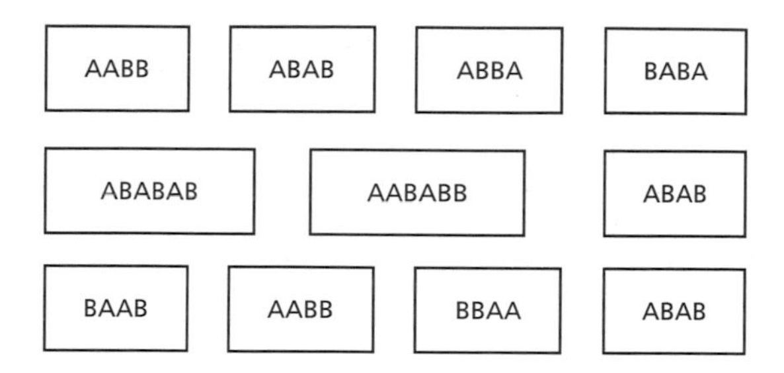

Figure 7.4 Randomized permuted blocks.

Stratified randomization

Here, the eligible population is stratified (*divided*) according to a minimal number of important prognostic factors, such as gender, race or centre (*multi-centre trial*), etc., before randomizing subjects within each stratum to the compared groups of a clinical trial. This is done in order to ensure a balance of the stratification factors through the compared groups e.g. age groups.

Randomized consent method

This method is employed by trials interested in the efficacies of compared treatments as well as the effects of informed consent on treatment efficacy. It is also used in some clinical trials to lessen the effect of some patients' refusal to participate. Randomized consent methods are illustrated in Figure 7.5. Here, it is important to note that the important comparison to be made in the trial are between groups I and II, and not between treatments A and B.

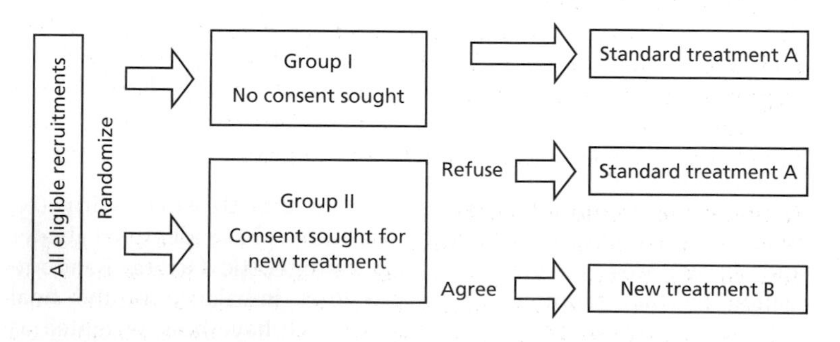

Figure 7.5 Randomized consent.

ADAPTIVE RANDOMIZATION METHODS

With adaptive methods the probability of being allocated to any group within the study is not fixed throughout the recruitment and randomization process. In fact, such allocation probabilities are adjusted as the trial progresses in order to correct any imbalances in the numbers of subjects within subgroups, or in response to the outcome data being obtained from the ongoing trial.

'Play the winner'

With this adaptive randomization method, the first subject is allocated by a simple randomization procedure and thereafter; every subsequent allocation is based on the success or failure of the immediate predecessor subject (Figure 7.6). Therefore, every subject is allocated to the treatment that his immediate predecessor received if success was recorded or they are allocated to the alternative treatment if failure was recorded in the immediate predecessor subject.

Figure 7.6 'Playing the winner' method. X-axis represents the sequence of patient allocation to treatment groups. ✓ means 'treatment success', × means 'treatment failure'.

Minimization

Minimisation is the most commonly used adaptive method of randomization. It involves identifying a few important prognostic factors in a trial and then applying a weighting system to them. Every subsequent subject is then randomized to the treatment group that would cause the least imbalance to the overall distribution of weighted prognostic factors between the compared groups. Minimization is performed in order to ensure an overall balance in the distribution of the more important prognostic factors between the various treatment groups of a trial.

Example: How minimization works

A clinical trial is conducted to compare a new anti-Alzheimer's drug (N) to a standard drug (S) in the elderly. The authors have identified gender and disease stage as being important prognostic factors. Randomization by minimization can ensure least imbalance in the final distribution of these prognostic factors which have been weighted as follows.

Prognostic factors	Ascribed weighting
Gender	1
Disease stage	2

So far into the trial, 100 recruitments have been randomized, as follows.

Factors	Drug N	Drug S	Imbalance	Weighted imbalance
Male	12	3	9	9
Female	38	47	9	9
Early stage dementia	39	32	7	14
Mid-stage dementia	11	18	7	14

Imagine that the 101st recruit was a male subject with mid-stage dementia:

If he were allocated to Drug N	If he were allocated to Drug S
Male subject imbalance increased to 10	Male subject imbalance reduced to 8
Weighted imbalance $(10 \times 1) = 10$	Weighted imbalance $(8 \times 1) = 8$
Mid-stage dementia imbalance reduced to 6	Mid-stage dementia imbalance increased to 8
Weighted imbalance $(6 \times 2) = 12$	Weighted imbalance $(8 \times 2) = 16$
Overall weighted imbalance $= 10 + 12 = 22$	Overall weighted imbalance $= 8 + 16 = 24$

Therefore, in order to minimize overall imbalance in the distribution of prognostic factors between compared groups, subject 101 would be randomized to receive Drug N i.e. accepting an imbalance of 22 instead of Drug S which would mean an imbalance of 24. Minimization becomes impractical when more than 3–4 prognostic factors are involved.

Interim analyses

This describes the analysis of trial results that are performed at predetermined time points before the conclusion of a clinical trial. Interim analyses are performed so as to identify early from the data gathered up until such points, significantly beneficial (or harmful!) effects of one treatment over another. The motivation for this procedure is to avoid further disadvantage to those subjects allocated to the apparently inferior treatment(s). Interim analyses also allow researchers to identify and correct any flaws in the trial process that may otherwise go unnoticed.

The trouble with checking repeatedly, however, is that sooner or later, a false-positive finding will occur (after all, even a $p < 0.05$ carries a

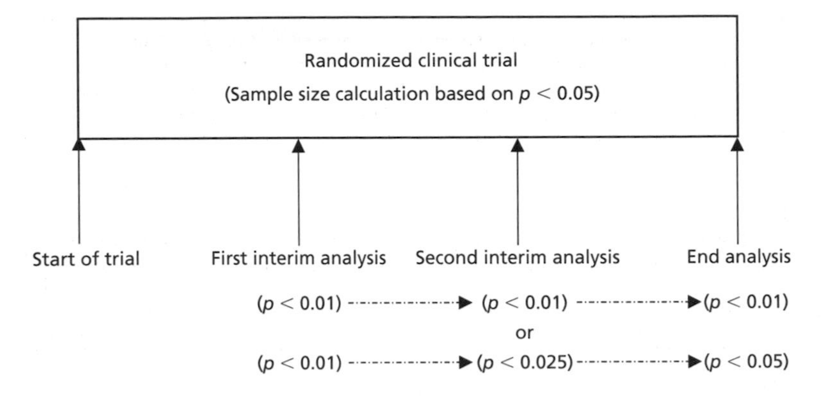

Figure 7.7 Interim analysis.

one in 20 risk of such a Type I error!). Another potential source of such Type I errors comes from the fact that in an ongoing trial, only a part of the required sample size would have been recruited at the time points that interim analyses are carried out.

In order to guard against a Type I error, interim analyses should be subject to a strict 'group sequential' trial protocol with:

- More stringent significance criteria than planned (e.g. $p < 0.01$), right until the end of the trial. This is to correct for the smaller than required sample sizes at the interim points. Remember that the original sample size calculation would have been based on a larger p-value (e.g. $p < 0.05$) or
- Smaller p-values in the earlier interim analyses, adjusting (increasing) the p-values accordingly as the sample size increases in the later interim analyses (Figure 7.7).

(See specialized text on clinical trials for details.)

Factorial designs

Factorial study designs are used in RCTs where two or more treatment factors are being compared simultaneously (Figure 7.8). Here, subjects are allocated to different treatment groups featuring different combinations of the treatment factors. Unless an outright placebo group is included in a factorial design, only relative comparisons can be made between the groups involved.

A randomized trial is set up to compare different modes of surgical drainage in the reduction of post-operative complications following mastectomy. The treatment factors of interest in this study are the location of post-operative drainage and the use of post-operative suction. The four treatment groups in the trail had different combinations of factors as follows:

I	II	III	IV
Drain through surgical incision & No suction	Drain through surgical incision & Suction	Drain through separate incision & No suction	Drain through separate incision & Suction

Figure 7.8 Example of a factorial design clinical trial.

Therefore, from the factorial design decribed in Figure 7.8, it would be impossible to draw any inferences about the absolute benefits of post-operative surgical drainage or post-operative suction. In order to make such comparisons, 'drainage versus non-drainage' or 'suction versus non-suction' groups would need to be explicitly compared, that is, a matter for another kind of trial. This is an error that is encountered frequently when assessing the results of a factorial design clinical trial.

Cross-over designs

Treatments being received in the groups of a study are 'switched' after a specified period (Figure 7.9). At the end of the study, data on each subject whilst on the different treatments (*paired data!*) are then compared for each study participant. The advantage of this method is that each individual acts as his control. There can be no better control than one's own self. The main disadvantage, however, is that the effects of treatment can be carried over from one treatment period to another.

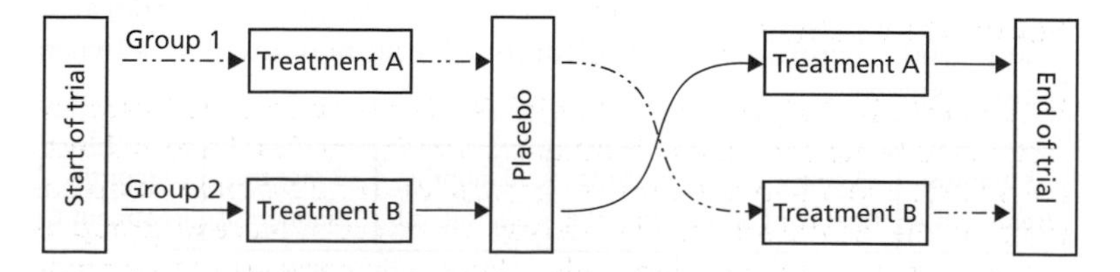

Figure 7.9 Cross-over trial design.

Cluster randomization designs

In these RCTs, actual treatment centres and not individual subjects are randomized to the respective allocated treatments. All the subjects in a centre therefore receive the same treatment to which that centre was allocated (Figure 7.10).

Cluster randomization is particularly useful in trials where it would be impractical to blind clinicians to the nature of treatments that the subjects have received, such as when making comparisons between a surgical intervention and a medical intervention.

They are also useful whenever compared treatments are of such a nature that any single centre cannot reasonably be expected to switch between the allocated treatment interventions. Examples include trials making comparisons between different psychotherapies, or different health education or health-promotion programmes, etc.

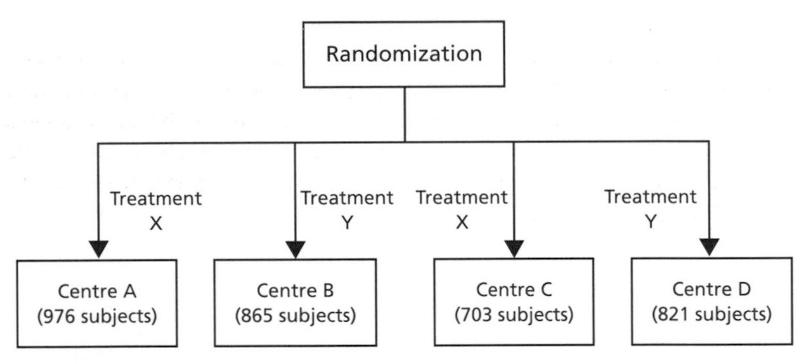

Figure 7.10 Cluster design.

n-of-1 trials

In this type of study, competing treatments are randomized to different time periods for each trial subject. Each subject is then administered the respective treatments (including placebo) sequentially over allocated time periods (Figure 7.11). A typical *n*-of-1 trial may involve between 1 and 30 subjects.

3 months	3 months	3 months	3 months	3 months	3 months
Treatment A	Treatment B	Treatment C	Treatment B	Treatment A	Treatment C

Figure 7.11 Treatment allocation for a subject in an *n*-of-1 trial.

- Preferably double-blind, the object of this type of trial is to enable an individual patient to identify a treatment period that corresponded with the most subjective benefit.
- *n*-of-1 studies are particularly useful for studies involving chronic symptoms, such as chronic pain, where subjective ratings of severity make more clinical sense than an objective measure.
- *n*-of-1 trials are only appropriate with conditions whose pathologies are relatively stable over a long periods. A disease condition that improves or worsens over the trial period would confound the results of an *n*-of-1 study. This is because symptoms will alter with disease changes.
- Although hopefully improving the severity of symptoms experienced by subjects, the treatments being compared in an *n*-of-1 study should not directly alter the underlying disease process itself. Worsening or improvement of underlying pathological processes would cause a change in symptom severity, which would also confound the results of such a trial.

A Hawthorne effect is commonly observed in the subjects of an *n*-of-1 study during the initial phase. This effect, however, is not often sustained, producing improvements in symptoms only during the early stages. Such phenomena can bias the results of an *n*-of-1 study. Furthermore, carry-over effects from one treatment period to another can also occur, resulting in a distortion of results.

Open trials

With open clinical trials, a required sample size is not specified at the start. Instead, the other components of the sample size formula, that is, significance level, required power and a would-be acceptable effect size, are defined before the start of the trial. As subjects are then recruited into the trial, accumulated data are inspected continually or periodically until the pre-specified trial end-point conditions are met. Conditions needing to be fulfilled at this trial end-point would consist of a pre-stated minimal acceptable effect size occurring at the predefined significance level and power. The sample size (n) of an open trial is therefore subject to achieving a desired effect size (δ) at the predefined α and β conditions (see Figure 7.12 and Figure 7.13).

Remember:

$$n \geqslant \frac{2\sigma^2(\varepsilon_{\alpha/2} + \varepsilon_\beta)^2}{\delta^2}$$

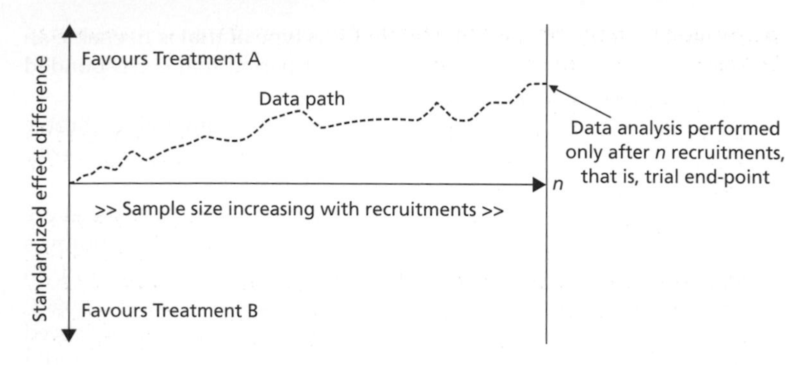

Figure 7.12 Closed-plan trials.

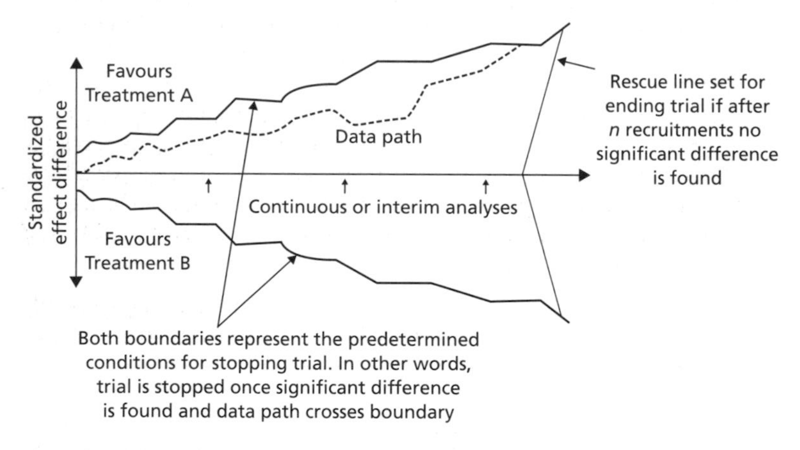

Figure 7.13 Open-plan trials.

n = number of subjects required in each group; σ = standard deviation of property; α = significance level (e.g. if $\alpha = 0.05$ then $\alpha/2 = 0.025$ and $\alpha/2 = 1.96$; $\beta = 1 -$ power (e.g. if power = 0.9 then $\beta = 0.1$ and $\beta = 1.282$); δ = estimated size of difference or effect.

Non-randomized clinical trials

NON-RANDOMIZED TRIALS WITH CONCURRENT CONTROL SUBJECTS

With these studies, treatment groups are compared concurrently. However, allocation to the different treatment groups of a trial is not performed via a proper randomization process. Instead, allocation may be based on other criteria, such as:

- Alternate A B A B A B ... allocation.
- Allocation by geographically defined areas – subjects from certain areas are given Treatment A, whereas those from other areas are given Treatment B.
- Cluster allocation (not cluster randomization!), for example by hospital, where Treatment A is allocated to all subjects in one hospital and Treatment B is allocated to all subjects in another hospital. Cluster allocations are also often performed on the basis of GP practice where subjects belonging to certain practices are given Treatment A and those from other practices are given Treatment B.
- Allocation by address, for example odd and even number addresses, where subjects with odd address numbers are given Treatment A and those with even address numbers are given Treatment B.
- Allocation by vital data, for example date of birth. This may involve subjects born between January and June being given Treatment A, whereas those born between July and December are given Treatment B. Other examples include the use of surnames as the basis of allocation. Here, subjects whose surnames start with letters A–M may be given Treatment A, whereas those with surnames starting with N–Z are given Treatment B.

Obviously, these methods of treatment allocation, although possibly easier or cheaper to perform, inevitably introduce many kinds of bias into a clinical trial and should not be considered.

HISTORICAL CONTROL SUBJECTS

Historical control subjects can occasionally be used in the methodologies of 'unrandomized' clinical trials. Here, in order to make comparisons between treatment interventions, experimental subjects with a specific disorder are compared with similar control subjects drawn from the past, when control interventions were administered.

The use of historical controls in unrandomized clinical trials offers some advantages. A ready access to the large amounts of data that have been gathered over several years reduces the costs involved in conducting such (potentially large) studies. Historical control subjects are also useful in studies where the control interventions are regarded as being no longer ethical, too costly or too impractical to administer in the setting of a randomized trial.

However, the use of historical control subjects also presents numerous problems. First, any systematic differences in outcomes found between current experimental subjects and historical control subjects may be due to the different time eras when subjects were treated and not the compared treatments themselves, that is, time-related confounding factor.

Furthermore, these historical control subjects may not have been in a clinical trial themselves at the time, resulting in a one-sided Hawthorne effect enjoyed by the current experimental subjects. Lack of proper clinical trial conditions in the historical control subjects can also mean that there were vague or poorly defined inclusion and exclusion criteria for these subjects at the time. Blinding procedures are not feasible when using historical control subjects and therefore the potential for observer bias is high.

For all these reasons, historical controls should only be used as a last resort.

What do the results show?

The measures discussed in the prospective studies section (Chapter 6), such as relative risk, relative risk reduction, relative risk increase, absolute risk reduction, absolute risk increase and others, are all applicable to RCTs. Of particular relevance to RCTs, however, are the issues of number-needed-to-treat (NNT) and number-needed-to-harm (NNH). Both are discussed in more detail here.

Understanding of NNT begins with a calculation of absolute risk reduction (ARR). According to the example used earlier (p. 110), where two vaccines, A and B, were tested on two similar populations and were reported as reducing the risk of influenza (*outcome*) in the elderly:

Vaccine A	No influenza	Influenza	Total
Exposed (V)	600,000	400,000	1,000,000
Control	200,000	800,000	1,000,000
Total	800,000	1,200,000	2,000,000

Vaccine B	No influenza	Influenza	Total
Exposed (V)	999,960	40	1,000,000
Control	999,920	80	1,000,000
Total	1,999,880	120	2,000,000

ARR = p2 − p1

ARR using Vaccine A
= 0.8 − 0.4
= 0.4

ARR using Vaccine B
= 0.00008 − 0.00004
= 0.00004

Number-needed-to-treat (NNT)

NNT can be defined, as the number of patients required to be treated with a therapeutic factor for the stated treatment duration in order to achieve the desired outcome in one patient. NNT is calculated by reciprocating absolute risk reduction (ARR).

$$\text{NNT} = 1/\text{ARR}$$

Therefore, respective NNT for vaccines A and B would be:

Vaccine A

$$\begin{aligned} \text{ARR} &= 0.4 \\ \text{NNT} &= 1/0.4 \\ &= 2.5 \text{ (rounded up to 3)} \end{aligned}$$

Vaccine B

$$\begin{aligned} \text{ARR} &= 0.00004 \\ \text{NNT} &= 1/0.00004 \\ &= 25{,}000 \end{aligned}$$

(Note: NNT is always rounded 'upwards' to whole numbers! For example, 1.2 is rounded up to 2.)

Clearly, from the above illustration it is understandable NNT as a measure is profoundly more popular amongst researchers and clinicians alike. The principal attraction lies in its simplicity and digestibility when compared with measures such as ARR.

A drug with NNT of *n* implies that on average *n* patients have to be treated for the stated treatment duration in order to achieve a beneficial outcome in one patient … simple!

Furthermore, because an element of treatment duration is included in determining NNT, an idea of real treatment cost is conveyed to the clinician.

COMPARING RRR, ARR AND NNT INTERPRETATIONS OF THE SAME RESULT

- NNT: according to the results, three children would need to be treated with Vaccine A in order to prevent one case of influenza, whereas 25,000 children would need to be treated with Vaccine B in order to prevent one case of influenza. Doctors, nurses, managers, politicians, scientists and the general public would all sooner relate to facts presented in this NNT format than in the following ARR format.
- ARR: according to the results, Vaccine A achieved an 0.40 reduction in the absolute risk of influenza compared with the 0.00004 reduction achieved with Vaccine B. Compare this to the potentially misleading RRR format.

- RRR: according to the results, both Vaccine A and Vaccine B achieved a 50% reduction in the risk of influenza.

Number-needed-to-harm (NNH)

NNH is similar in concept to NNT. NNH is defined as the number of patients needed to be exposed to a therapeutic factor for the stated treatment duration in order to achieve a harmful outcome in one patient. An example of such harmful outcome could be secondary hypothyroidism in patients on long-term lithium therapy.

NNH is calculated by reciprocating 'absolute risk increase' (ARI):

$$\text{NNH} = 1/\text{ARI}$$

(Note: NNH is rounded 'downwards' to whole numbers!)

RISK–BENEFIT ANALYSIS

To treat or not to treat, that is the question.

The NNT and NNH values associated with a particular treatment can be compared in a risk–benefit analysis in order to justify the administration of that treatment to an individual patient. The example below illustrates how this is done.

EXAMPLE

The results of a large RCT conducted over a year have just been published. A new wonder-drug 'Packitin' was compared with an established anti-psychotic drug regarding therapeutic efficacy in treatment-resistant schizophrenia.

In this trial, 2000 treatment-resistant schizophrenia cases were randomized into two groups. One group received Packitin and the other received the established anti-psychotic drug, Bolzar. Both drugs were administered at equivalent dosages.

The outcome measures used in the trial for therapeutic effectiveness was a 60% reduction in both positive and negative symptom scores on the PANSS questionnaire at the end of the one-year period. Scores on this questionnaire were recorded at the beginning of the trial, at three-monthly intervals and at the end of the trial.

Assuming complete follow-up and a zero drop-out rate, consider the results tabulated below which, incidentally, also include recorded rates of irreversible alopecia (a recognized side-effect of Packitin) observed during the trial, amongst experimental group subjects.

Drug	Effective	Non-effective	Alopecia	Total
Packitin	600	400	7	1000
Bolzar	200	800	0	1000

Risk of continued treatment resistance with Packitin:

$$\begin{aligned} p1 &= 400/1000 \\ &= 0.4 \end{aligned}$$

Risk of continued treatment resistance with Bolzar:

$$\begin{aligned} p2 &= 800/1000 \\ &= 0.8 \\ \text{ARR} &= p2 - p1 \\ &= 0.4 \\ \text{NNT} &= 1/0.4 \\ &= 2.5 \text{ (rounded up to 3)} \end{aligned}$$

In other words, you need to treat three treatment-resistant schizophrenic patients with Packitin for one year in order to achieve a 60% reduction in positive and negative symptoms in one patient.

Risk of developing alopecia with Packitin:

$$\begin{aligned} p1 &= 7/1000 \\ &= 0.007 \end{aligned}$$

Risk of developing alopecia with Bolzar:

$$\begin{aligned} p2 &= 0 \\ \text{ARI} &= p1 - p2 \\ &= 0.007 \\ \text{NNH} &= 1/0.007 \\ &= 142.9 \text{ (rounded up to 143)} \end{aligned}$$

In other words, you need to treat 143 treatment-resistant schizophrenic patients with Packitin for one year in order for irreversible alopecia to occur in one patient.

You are faced with a clinical dilemma because whilst considering commencing a treatment-resistant schizophrenic patient of yours on Packitin you are concerned about the possibility of irreversible alopecia. Your patient is a 31-year-old single lady! What is the likelihood that Packitin would benefit this patient (*effective control of symptoms*) as opposed to harm her (*hair loss!*)? The likelihood of benefit compared with the likelihood of harm can be calculated by comparing the reciprocal of NNT (ARR) with that of NNH (ARI).

Benefit versus Harm
= 1/NNT (ARR) versus 1/NNH (ARI)
= 0.4 versus 0.007, that is
= 57 : 1 in favour of treatment with Packitin

Your dilemma is not over. The cost of alopecia to your patient (being a young, single, female and being particularly fond of her hair) you estimate at being four times that of the 'average' patient involved in the RCT. By incorporating this into the decision-making process the benefit versus harm equation becomes:

= 1/NNT (ARR) versus 1/NNH (ARI) × 4
= 0.4 versus 0.028, that is
= 14 : 1 in favour of treatment with Packitin

Furthermore, tormenting auditory hallucinations particularly incapacitate your patient and you estimate the impact on her quality of life at being twice that of the 'average' patient involved in the RCT. Incorporating this into the decision-making process, the benefit versus harm equation becomes:

= 1/NNT (ARR) × 2 versus 1/NNH (ARI) × 4
= 0.8 versus 0.028, that is
= 29 : 1 in favour of treatment with Packitin

Therefore, in the final analysis, this lady with treatment-resistant schizophrenia is 29 times more likely to benefit from, than be harmed by, treatment with Packitin.

As illustrated above, the risk–benefit analysis of any treatment can be individualized to suit the circumstances and needs of any particular patient by appropriately adjusting the likelihood of benefit (ARR) or likelihood of harm (ARI) values.

CALCULATING THE 95% CONFIDENCE INTERVAL FOR AN NNT VALUE

$$\text{95\% CI of NNT} = \frac{1}{\text{ARR} \pm 1.96\sqrt{\dfrac{\text{p2} \times (1-\text{p2})}{n_{\text{control}}} + \dfrac{\text{p1} \times (1-\text{p1})}{n_{\text{experimental}}}}}$$

How do the results affect the care of my patients?

This step is concerned with how applicable the results of an RCT are to the care of patients and how they may (if at all) change your practice.

Even when an RCT fulfils all the validity criteria and has shown an appreciable beneficial effect with an experimental treatment, questions still have to be asked by clinicians, such as:

- Ensure that the subjects who participated in the RCT are not essentially different from your patients.
- There may be implications for your practice if the area of healthcare examined by a RCT is directly relevant to the patients in your care.
- Would the said treatment confer any added benefit (or harm) to your patients?
- What does your patient think about the said treatment in light of their beliefs, culture, etc.?
- Are they comfortable with the risk–benefit assessment as it applies to them?
- Is treatment accessible and affordable?

This is where your clinical judgement based on experience and expertise comes into play.

Handling survival time data

8

Introduction

This section deals with the critical appraisal of all kinds of studies presenting 'survival time' data. In these studies (most often randomized clinical trials), outcomes in the compared groups are measured in terms of the time elapsed before a particular end-point event occurs in the study subjects.

Survival time data

Examples can include 'time to death' or 'time to recovery' or 'time to complete wound healing' or 'time to second stroke event' or 'duration of hospital stay' or 'time to relapse' or any other specified end-point. The length of time from entering into a study to developing the end-point event is called the 'survival time'.

Figure 8.1 illustrates data on the start dates and survival times gathered on 10 subjects recruited into the treatment arm of a one-year major stroke randomized clinical trial.

Subjects A, G and I were recruited at the commencement of the study whilst the other subjects came in at a later stage as denoted by the start of the broken lines. The diamond shape represents the occurrence of the

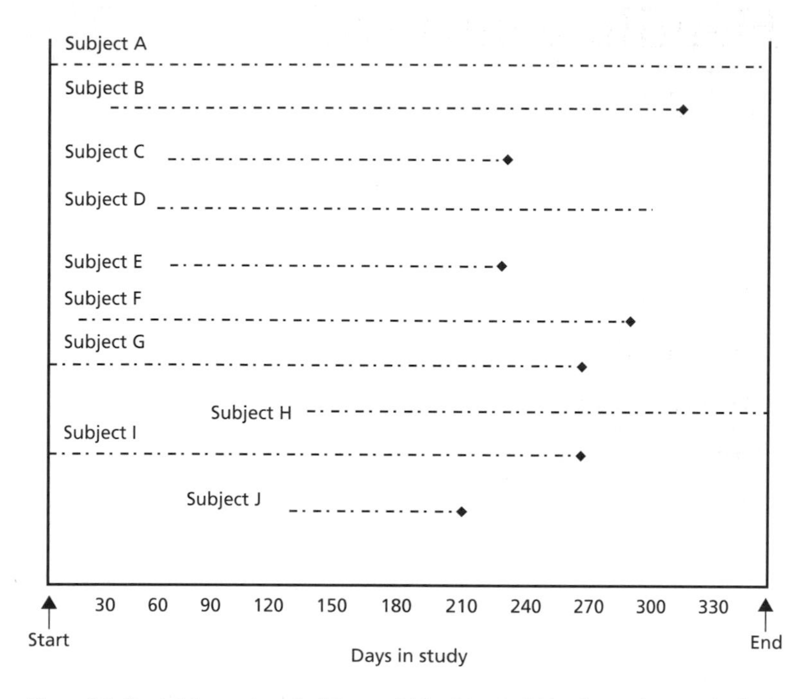

Figure 8.1 Start dates and survival times of 10 subjects with major stroke recruited into a one-year study.

end-point event, which in this case is death. However, start times are really unimportant in analysing this type of data. Of more relevance are the survival times of the subjects, which are summarized in Figure 8.2 with all start dates set to zero.

As is often the case, however, survival times on some subjects may be unobtainable (A, D and H) either because they do not achieve the end-point event by the end of the study or because they drop out of the study or are lost to follow-up, etc. This phenomenon of unobtainable data is known as 'censoring' and data on such subjects are denoted with a (+) sign. Incidentally, the time from entering into a study to becoming censored is termed a 'censored survival time'.

'Survival probability' describes the chance that an individual will not develop an end-point event over a given time duration. (Note: end-point probability = 1 − survival probability.) As shown in Figure 8.2, by day 91 of the study, one subject had developed the end-point event

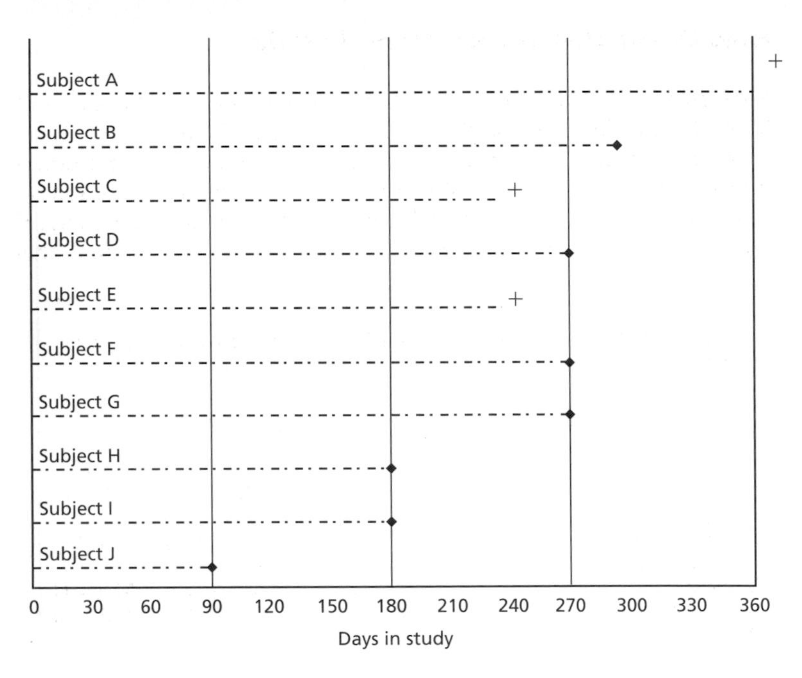

Figure 8.2 Survival times of 10 subjects recruited into a one-year study with all start times set to zero.

(*death*). Therefore, it may be said that in this study, the probability of survival for 90 days is 90% (9/10). Similarly, by day 181 in the study another two of the remaining nine subjects had died, making the probability of survival for 180 days 70% (7/10).

By day 271, another three subjects had died and, significantly, two subjects had also been censored. Though the initial temptation may be to calculate the 270-day survival based on the 'four deaths out of 10 subjects' formula, this would be an error!

The probability of survival for 270 days *cannot* be calculated in the same way as was done for 90 and 180 days because of the two censored subjects whose survival data cannot be determined. In other words, it is unknown whether these two subjects would have been alive or dead, had they remained in the study for 270 days.

In order to overcome the problem posed by censoring when calculating survival probabilities, a clever procedure called the 'Kaplan–Meier method', which estimates a cumulative survival probability, is used instead.

How the Kaplan–Meier method works

First, survivial probabilities are *only* calculated whenever the event of interest occurs in a study and at no other time (see Table 8.1).

Second, whenever an event occurs, survival probabilities are determined in the following way. The survival probability just prior to that event is brought forward and adjusted using the post-event survival rate of the remaining uncensored subjects (see Table 8.1). It is this

Table 8.1 Survival life table of 10 experimental-group subjects in a one-year major stroke study

	Number censored	Number at risk	Number of deaths	Numbers remaining	Kaplan–Meier calculation	Cumulative survival probability
Start	–	10	0	10	NA	100% (1)
By day 90	–	10	1	9	100% × (9/10)	90% (0.9)
By day 180	–	9	2	7	90% × (7/9)	70% (0.7)
By day 240	2	–	–	–	–	–
By day 270	–	5	3	2	70% × (2/5)	60% (0.6)
By day 300	–	2	1	1	60% × (1/2)	30% (0.3)
By day 360	1	–	–	–	–	–

Number of cases: 10; censored: 3; events: 7; NA = not applicable.

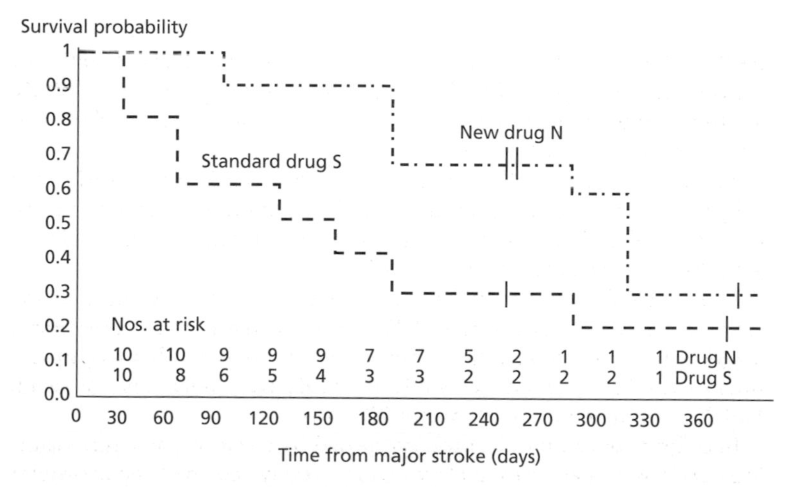

Figure 8.3 Kaplan–Meier survival curve of one-year major stroke randomized clinical trial comparing new drug with standard treatment.

repeated carrying over of survival probabilities that creates a cumulative survival probability.

Kaplan–Meier survival curve

All survival time data are usually plotted on a Kaplan–Meier survival curve such as the one shown in Figure 8.3. The example used below is of a one-year randomized clinical study, comparing the efficacies of a new drug and a standard drug in the acute treatment phase following diagnosis with a major stroke event. The study had 10 subjects each in the treatment and control groups.

Median survival time

Generally, survival times are not felt to obey a normal distribution. This, along with the problem posed by censored observations is the reason why a 'median' measure (non-parametric measure) is used to summarize and describe survival time data and not a 'mean' measure.

The 'median survival time' is defined as the time duration from the start of a study that coincides with a 0.5 (50%) probability of survival. In other words, the median survival time represents the time taken in a study for half the subjects to have an event (Figure 8.4). It can be determined on the Kaplan–Meier survival curve by visually tracing the time value on

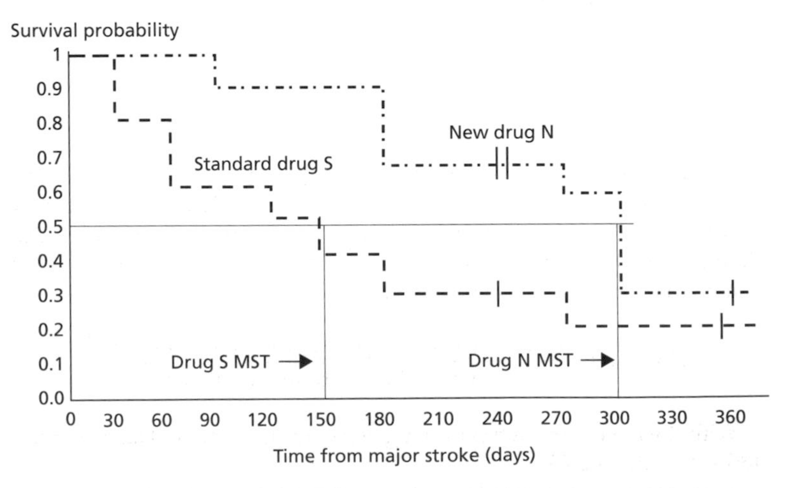

Figure 8.4 Respective median survival times of subjects on Drug S and new Drug N. MST = median survival time.

the curve corresponding to a 0.5 probability of survival. Naturally, median survival times are usually presented with *p*-values and confidence intervals.

From the illustration above, it can be concluded that newly diagnosed patients with major stroke would have a median survival time of 300 days if treated with new drug (N) compared with 150 days on standard treatment drug (S). Naturally, these figures would be presented with the appropriate *p*-values and confidence intervals in study reports. Note that median survival time cannot be estimated for as long as survival remains above 0.5.

Note: the chance that an individual will not achieve the end-point event within a given duration in a study has already been described as the 'survival probability' (see p. 147). Similarly, chance that an individual will achieve the end-point event within a given duration in a study can be described as the 'end-point probability' (1 − Survival probability).

Therefore, by 180 days into the study, seven subjects out of 10 remained and the end-point event had occurred in three subjects:

Survival probability in 180 days = 0.7 (70%)
End-point probability in 180 days = 1 − 0.7
= 0.3 (30%)

The 'Log-rank test' statistical test used when comparing survival time data. It computes a *p*-value that answers the following question: 'If no difference really existed between the compared interventions, what is the probability of getting survival curves or median survival times as discrepant as those observed?'

Hazard

Hazard is defined as the instantaneous probability of an end-point event in a study, that is, the probability that an individual will have an end-point event at a given time (t). Hazard is the underlying factor that determines the occurrence or non-occurrence of an end-point event and can be calculated according to the formula:

$$\text{Hazard} = \frac{\text{Instantaneous end-point probability at time (t)}}{\text{Survival probability at time (t)}}$$

With the major stroke treatment group example above, Hazard at day 180 = 0.3/0.7 = 0.43.

A hazard of 0.43 means that in the treatment group of the major stroke study, the instantaneous probability of death on day 180 for any of the subjects was 43%. *This is not to be confused with the end-point probability, which describes the chance of achieving the end-point event within 180 days from the start of the study.*

The advantages of hazard in survival time analyses are two-fold. First, the process underpinning survival or event in a study can be better understood by observing a hazard plot that shows hazard changes over time (Table 8.2). Second, by assuming proportionally varying hazards, a hazard ratio (similar to relative risk) can be derived by comparing the hazard functions of two or more groups (Figure 8.5).

Table 8.2 Hazard function in treatment and control groups on the day's end-point-event occurred

Time (t)	Day 30	Day 60	Day 90	Day 120	Day 150	Day 180	Day 270	Day 300
Hazard (N)	–	–	0.1	–	–	0.43	0.66	2.33
Hazard (S)	0.25	0.66	–	1	1.5	2.33	4	–

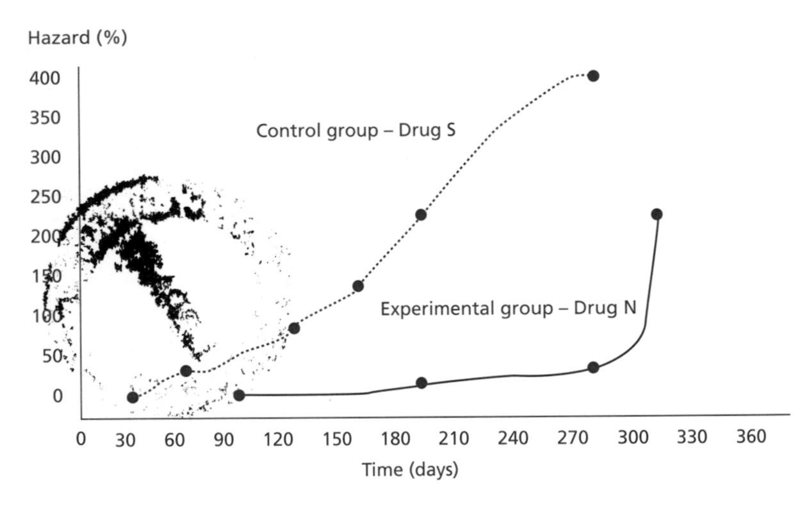

Figure 8.5 Graphical comparison on hazard function in both groups of the one-year major stroke study.

Hazard ratio

Comparing corresponding hazard values between two groups produces a hazard ratio, which is defined as the relative risk of an instantaneous end-point event in one group compared with another group.

An assumption must be made in the determination of hazard ratios. Using the hazard values on day 180 from the above example, the hazard ratio can be calculated as follows:

$$\begin{aligned}\text{Hazard ratio} &= \text{Hazard Drug N}/\text{Hazard Drug S}\\ &= 0.43/2.33\\ &= 0.2\end{aligned}$$

This means subjects on new Drug N appeared to be around five times less likely to die than subjects on standard treatment Drug S in the one-year study. Note however that only 10 subjects were involved in this illustrative study, and hence the difference in hazards is not likely to be a significant one.

Critical appraisal of systematic reviews

9

Introduction

A systematic review is a scientific evaluation of several studies that have been conducted on a specific clinical question. By pooling together the results from several studies, the evidence drawn from systematic reviews can be very powerful and influential indeed. Unsurprisingly therefore, systematic reviews are regarded as a gold standard source of research evidence, even more so than individual randomized clinical trials.

Systematic reviews

Systematic reviews are mostly conducted on randomized trials, but can also be conducted on other types of studies, including non-randomized trials, observational studies and even diagnostic test studies where several ROC plots are summarized in order to increase the precision of a test (*sensitivity and specificity values*).

A systematic review typically starts with the definition and refinement of a clinical problem. Having carved out a precise clinical question, researchers then devise an explicit and objective protocol on how the systematic review is to be conducted.

This protocol usually includes all aspects of the proposed systematic review, including methodology, search strategies, inclusion and exclusion criteria, other validity criteria for included studies and instruments to be used in the review for extracting data such as data extraction sheets, checklists, etc. The proposed methodology for the meta-analysis calculation and other statistical issues are also specified in the protocol of a systematic review. In other words, this pre-prepared protocol becomes the 'Holy Grail' of a systematic review, stating how most things are to be done in the review.

The next step in a systematic review is usually to perform a comprehensive search in order to identify studies been that have conducted on the clinical subject concerned. The search for both published and unpublished studies should be thorough and exhaustive and should include all relevant local and international sources such as databases and journals, reference lists, registers of studies, ethics committee registers, etc.

Following the search process, researchers conducting a systematic review would hopefully have identified a number of studies conducted round and about a particular clinical subject. Researchers then proceed to apply inclusion and exclusion criteria as specified in the protocol to these identified studies.

For example, inclusion criteria may specify 'clinical trials conducted on bulimia nervosa, examining the efficacy of any anti-depressants in the relief of binge and purge symptoms' as the basis for accepting studies into a review, whereas factors such as 'non-randomization or a less than three-month follow-up duration' may be listed as exclusion criteria.

In most systematic reviews, two or three independent assessors would apply the inclusion and exclusion criteria, thereby ensuring a necessary degree of objectivity. Most protocols would also state how any disagreements are to be dealt with, as well as the minimum degree of inter-rater agreement necessary for inclusion into the review. All studies considered are therefore subject to the same degree of scrutiny, thereby reducing the chance of selection bias in the systematic review.

Having applied the inclusion and exclusion criteria, studies deemed eligible are accepted whilst those that fall short of the selection criteria are noted, logged and excluded from the systematic review. Where necessary study authors can be contacted for clarification of unresolved issues about any particular studies.

From the studies that pass the tests described above, data are extracted strictly by use of the methods and instruments as stipulated in the protocol. This is to reduce the chance of observer bias. Extracted data usually concern issues such as randomization, sample size, follow-up duration, intention-to-treat analysis, size of effect, etc.

As an optional procedure, accepted studies may be assigned a weighting at this stage if relevant. Weighting is usually assigned based on the relative strengths (e.g. sample size, methodology, etc.) of the individual studies.

The methodology of systematic reviews should include a meta-analysis calculation. A meta-analysis calculation is usually performed as part of a systematic review so as to sum up the respective results of all the involved studies to produce an overall figure. Having carried out a weighting procedure, better quality studies can then be given more influence in the meta-analysis calculation from which the overall summary estimate is derived.

Meta-analysis

A meta-analysis is a statistical summation of the results from the studies that have been conducted on a specific clinical question. In other words, a meta-analysis pools the results from several studies to produce an overall estimate of the effect-size. Results are usually presented with *p*-values, confidence intervals and are displayed on a 'forest plot'.

Although details of meta-analysis calculations are beyond the scope of critical appraisal, it is worth noting that meta-analyses are also used to explore and analyse the various effects of random and systematic error that are seen to have occurred in the individual studies. A meta-analysis procedure ensures that these errors are identified and to an extent, adjusted and corrected prior to computing an overall estimate.

The outcome measure chosen to express effect size in a systematic review does not necessarily have to correspond to measures originally observed in the reviewed studies, which at any rate can vary from study to study. 'Absolute' measures (e.g. number-needed-to-treat, mean-effect-difference) or 'relative' measures (e.g. relative-risk, odds ratio) can equally be used to express effect size in a meta-analysis.

The results of a meta-analysis are usually displayed on a forest plot, as shown in Figure 9.1.

Elements of a forest plot (See Figure 9.1)

- The study column lists all the studies involved in the systematic review.
- The 'Experimental total' column contains the numbers of experimental subjects that participated in each study.

Meta-analysis of randomized clinical trials conducted on efficacy of nicotine-patch replacement therapy in smoking cessation

Study	NRT total	NRT cessation	Placebo total	Placebo cessation	OR (95% CI)
A et al.	1689	422	1678	118	3.56 (2.87–4.42)
B et al.	3658	358	3712	335	1.09 (0.94–1.28)
C et al.	804	289	753	73	5.23 (3.95–6.93)
D et al.	665	94	665	60	1.66 (1.18–2.34)
E et al.	2012	503	2019	444	1.18 (1.02–1.37)
F et al.	1253	163	1287	193	0.85 (0.68–1.06)

Test for heterogeneity: $\chi^2 = 145$, $df = 5$, $p = 0.6$
Overall odds ratio = 1.96 (95% CI 0.90–2.82)
Note: studies have not been weighted on this forest plot.

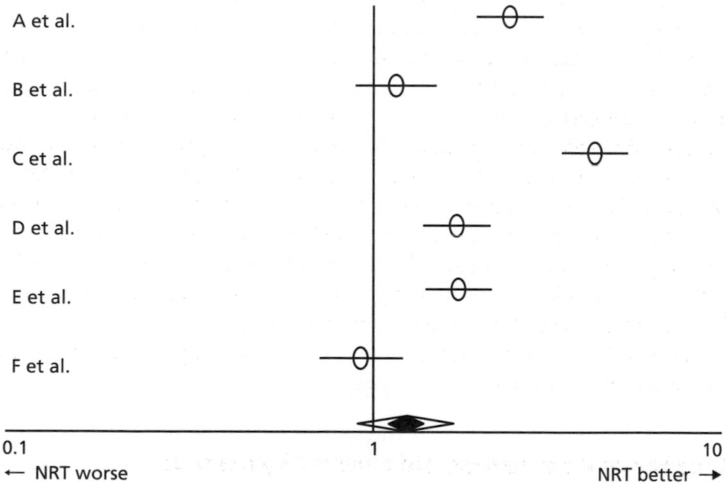

A et al.
B et al.
C et al.
D et al.
E et al.
F et al.

0.1 1 10
← NRT worse NRT better →

Figure 9.1 Homogeneity on a forest plot: *note that 'OR' dots have been deliberately made the same size for clarity.*

- The 'Experimental event' column states the number of events observed in each experimental group.
- The 'Control total' column contains the numbers of control subjects that participated in each study.
- The 'Control event' column states the number of events observed in each control group.
- The odds ratio (OR) derived from each study result can be ascribed a weighting based on certain criteria such as study sample size; on some forest plots, proportionately sized dots (or squares) may be used to represent the weighting ascribed to each study.
- The lines running across the 'OR' dot represent the confidence interval for that odds ratio.
- The midline of a forest plot corresponding to an odds ratio of '1' represents a 'no effect' line.
- Odds ratios with confidence intervals that cross the midline are regarded as non-significant. Furthermore, the farther away these are from the midline, the more significant the study findings are deemed to be.
- The solid diamond represents the overall OR estimate (1.86) of the studies presented in the meta-analysis. The outer encasing diamond represents the confidence interval of the overall odds ratio (95% CI 0.90–2.82).

Homogeneity and heterogeneity

In a meta-analysis of results from several studies, any variability seen to occur from study result to study result can be ascribed to chance, systematic differences or both.

ASCRIBED TO CHANCE

All reviewed studies have similar and consistent results; any observed differences are simply due to random variation. Such a collection of studies with non-significant between-study variability are said to have 'homogeneous' results.

ASCRIBED TO SYSTEMATIC DIFFERENCE

Real differences exist between the results of the reviewed studies even after allowing for random variation. Such a collection of disagreeable studies with significant between-study variability are said to have 'heterogeneous' results. The presence or absence of heterogeneity can be identified prior to a meta-analysis calculation by use of appropriate statistical tests such as the chi-square or the analysis of variance (ANOVA).

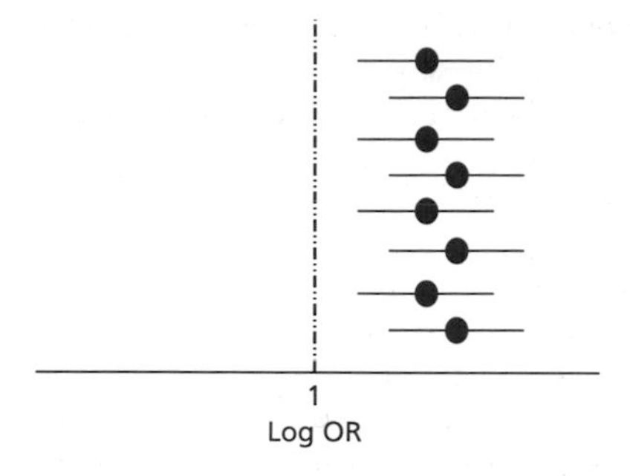

Figure 9.2 Forest plot: *note that 'OR' dots have been deliberately made the same size for clarity.*

'Homogeneity' is a term used in meta-analysis to describe non-significant variability between the results of examined studies. It is said to occur when the results of the respective studies are seen to broadly agree regarding the general magnitude and direction of effect (Figure 9.2).

The meta-analytic approach used when heterogeneity has been ruled out is called a 'fixed-effects model'. Here, weighting is simply assigned to each study based on either respective within-study variabilities or respective confidence intervals observed in each study. This is followed by a straightforward summary of results to give a pooled overall effect estimate.

'Heterogeneity' is a term used in a systematic review to describe a statistically significant inconsistency in results of examined studies. Heterogeneity occurs when the results of the represented studies disagree markedly on either the magnitude or direction of effect size.

When it occurs, heterogeneity should raise doubts about the respective methodologies of the involved studies and should prompt researchers to investigate the reasons for such discrepant results. Details of all these should be included in the systematic review report.

The meta-analytic approach used when heterogeneity exists is called a 'random-effects model'. Here, the observed between-study variability is also incorporated into the meta-analysis calculation prior to calculating a pooled overall effect estimate (Figure 9.3).

CAUSES OF HETEROGENEITY

Systematic differences in respective study results can be due to several subtle factors, including:

- Differences in respective methodologies, for example number of exclusion criteria.

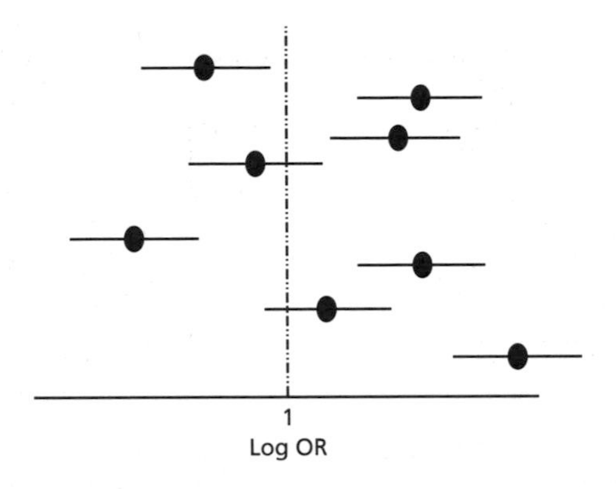

Figure 9.3 Heterogeneity on a forest plot: *note that 'OR' dots have been deliberately made the same size for clarity.*

- Differences in respective study population characteristics, for example ethnic groups or social class.
- Differences in the baseline risk of the respective populations studied.
- Differences in allocated treatment regimes or dosages.
- Differences in outcome measures, study end-points or follow-up durations.
- Differences in analytical methods, for example the chosen method for handling dropouts, or ITT.

Publication bias

This type of bias is particularly relevant to systematic reviews. It occurs because studies reporting positive findings are more likely to be accepted for publication in the journals than are studies (particularly small-sized ones) that report negative findings.

The search for studies to be included in a systematic review should therefore be as exhaustive as possible, including unpublished studies and those published in less-known journals, foreign publications, etc. Publication bias can be detected by constructing a 'funnel plot' of all identifiable studies that have been performed on a clinical subject.

FUNNEL PLOTS

Funnel plots work on the assumption that, if all studies conducted about a similar subject were represented graphically by plotting respective

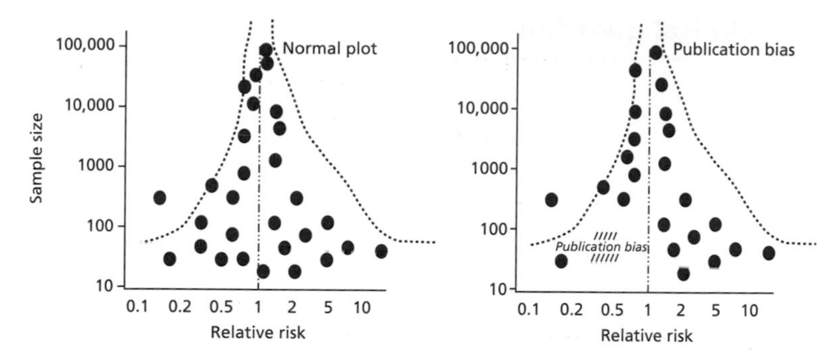

Figure 9.4 Funnel plot to detect publication bias. The funnel plot highlights the classic asymmetry that can result from publication bias where studies (especially small-sized ones) reporting negative findings are more likely to be unnoticed, unpublished and often vanish from all existence.

effect magnitudes against respective sample sizes, a funnel-shaped distribution would be formed. The funnel shape results from the fact that large studies generally have more precise results, which hardly vary about a mean estimate, whereas small studies generally have widely varying results about the mean estimate (Figure 9.4).

Therefore, the critical appraisal of a systematic review should ask the following:

- Is the study design methodologically sound?
- What do the results show?
- How do the results apply to the care of my patients?

Attempting to perform a summation of results, drawn from different studies carried out on different populations possibly from different countries and at different times can be a very scientifically delicate process. Systematic reviews can therefore prone to high degrees of bias if great care is not taken.

Because systematic reviews are the gold standard of medical evidence, flawed reviews can have a profoundly misleading effect on clinical practice. Therefore, readers should always subject systematic review reports to rigorous critical appraisal.

Is the study design methodologically sound?

The issues discussed below are the main considerations when assessing the strengths and weaknesses of systematic review methodology.

The clinical question

Critical appraisal of a systematic review should begin with a consideration of the primary clinical question being addressed and how relevant it is to your area of speciality.

The protocol

Formulation of an objective and explicit protocol at the outset of a systematic review provides guidance on the entire methodology of the review. This helps to minimize the chance of systematic errors that may arise from a variety of sources when conducting the review. A brief description of the protocol used in a systematic review should be provided in the review report.

The search

The search for eligible studies has to be thorough in order to reduce the chance of publication bias. Details of the search effort and specific details of attempts to counteract publication bias should be provided in the report of a systematic review.

Inclusion and exclusion criteria

The eligibility criteria applied to all studies identified from the search process should be clearly stated in the report of a systematic review, including definitions wherever applicable. The report should also describe the safeguards that were put in place to ensure that these criteria were applied objectively.

Inter-rater reliability

Usually, two or three assessors would independently pass judgements on the eligibility of studies to be included in a systematic review. The report of a systematic review should state the levels of inter-rater agreement on *all* the studies considered. Details should also be provided about how disagreements were handled. (See 'Inter-rater reliability' and 'Kappa statistic' in the Glossary of terms at the end of the book.)

Methodology of studies involved

The issue of randomization is paramount when assessing the methodologies of studies included in a systematic review. Randomization is a very powerful tool that guards against all kinds of biases and confounding factors. Therefore, systematic reviews that have included non-randomized studies should be regarded with caution because of the inevitably high risk of error!

Most respectable systematic reviews include only randomized studies in their study design. When non-randomized studies are included, these should be analysed separately.

Meta-analysis

A systematic review might include a meta-analysis calculation. Assumptions made in the meta-analysis calculation, as well as models (*fixed or random effects*) used in the determination of the overall effect estimate should be clearly stated and justified in a systematic review report.

Handling heterogeneity

In the report of a systematic review, attempts to identify heterogeneity should be stated along with the proposed explanations for any such observed heterogeneity. Whenever it is seen to exist, researchers should discuss the statistical manoeuvres employed in overcoming heterogeneity.

What do the results show?

The results of a meta-analysis are usually presented on a forest plot such as shown in Figure 9.5.

What observations can be made from the penicillin systematic review?

- The results are expressed in odds ratios, that is, the odds that therapeutic benefit (*outcome*) will be seen in the experimental group compared to that in the control group.
- From the forest plot, six of the 14 studies reviewed reported a beneficial effect. Most studies therefore found a beneficial effect on the

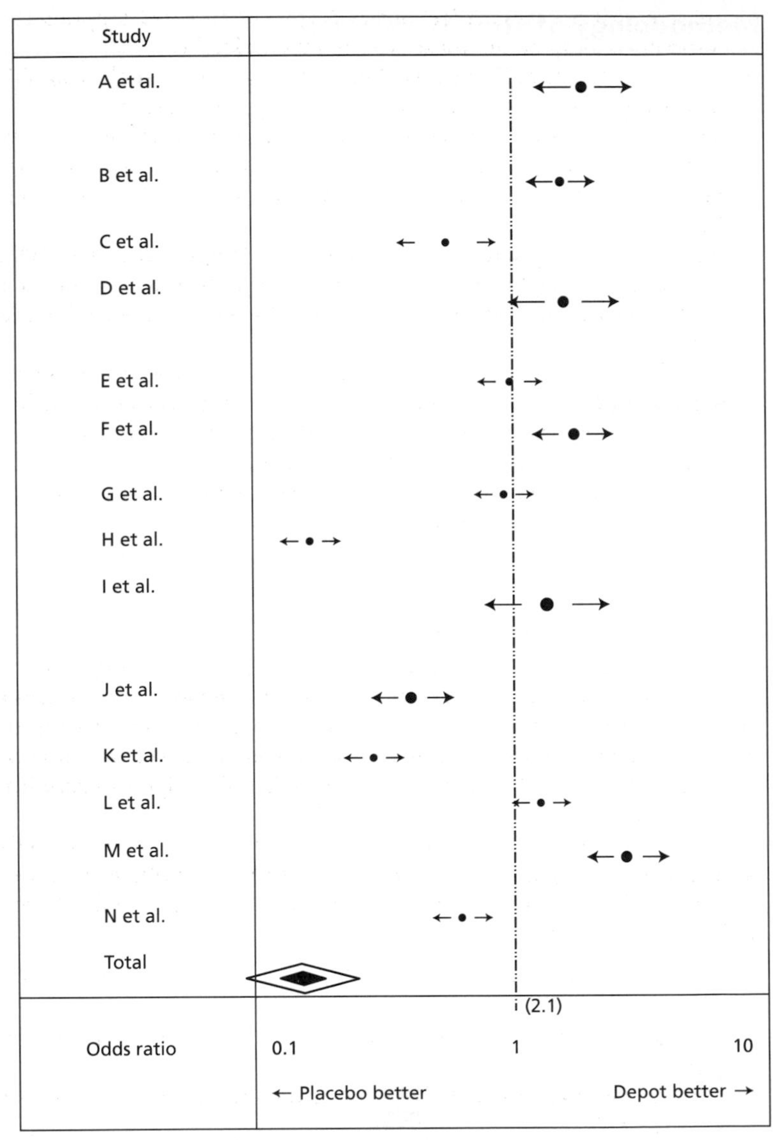

Test for heterogeneity: $\chi^2 = 145$, $df = 13$, $p < 0.05$

Overall OR (random effects) = 2.1 (0.8–3.4)

Figure 9.5 The results shown below are from a systematic review of 'randomized clinical trials' conducted on the efficacy of pre-operative penicillin in the prevention of post-operative infections following hip replacement surgery.

rates of post-operative infections in those who received prophylactic antibiotics compared to those who received placebo.

- In five studies, C et al., H et al., J et al., K et al. and N et al., a significantly better outcome was reported for the placebo group.
- The three studies, E et al., G et al. and I et al., reported statistically insignificant results, as reflected by their confidence intervals that cross the midline. In other words, no treatment performed better than the other.
- Results from the systematic review indicate heterogeneity at ($p < 0.05$).
- Studies conducted by D et al. and L et al. were only weakly significant as shown by the proximity to the midline of the respective confidence intervals.
- According to the meta-analysis, the overall effect estimate represented by a solid diamond suggests that prophylactic penicillin confers a beneficial effect on post-operative infection rates compared to placebo; odds-ratio of 2.1 (95% CI 0.8–3.4).
- The confidence interval of the overall effect estimate includes '1' and therefore a non-significant result.

How do the results apply to the care of my patients?

This step is concerned with how applicable the results of a systematic review are to the care of patients. Systematic reviews are the most powerful source evidence available, providing very precise estimates of treatment effects. This is because estimates are based on large amounts of data pooled from studies that have been subjected to rigorous scrutiny and weighting.

The risk–benefit analysis discussed in the randomized clinical trials section (Chapter 7) should also be performed with results from a systematic review because the same questions about applicability to the individual patient are still pertinent.

- Are the subjects used in the studies under review similar to my patients?
- Would the treatment confer any added benefit (or harm) to my patients?
- How do my patients feel about the treatment and the risk–benefit assessment?
- Is treatment accessible and affordable?

This is where your clinical judgement based on experience and expertise comes in.

Critical appraisal of clinical audit

10

Critical appraisal of clinical audit

Critical appraisal of clinical audits should begin by assessing the clinical importance of the practice area under examination (Figure 10.1).

Listed below are other considerations when assessing the strengths and weaknesses of clinical audits.

- Did the audit address a clinically important issue?
- Did the area of performance chosen for examination address the audit question?
- Were objective methods used for the measurement of performance?
- Were measured variable(s) a true reflection of performance?
- Were existing standards identified for that area of performance being measured?
- How did performance compare with standard?
- Were plausible explanations given for performance shortcomings (if any)?
- What recommendations were made to improve performance?
- Was audit cycle completed (re-audit)?

The following are additional considerations relevant to the critical appraisal of re-audit reports:

- What improvements were made in the re-audit design and methodology?
- How were the recommendations from previous audit implemented?
- Where there any difficulties impeding the implementation of the above recommendations?
- What steps were taken to overcome these constraints?
- What are re-audit recommendations?
- Go back to identifying existing standards for the area of performance

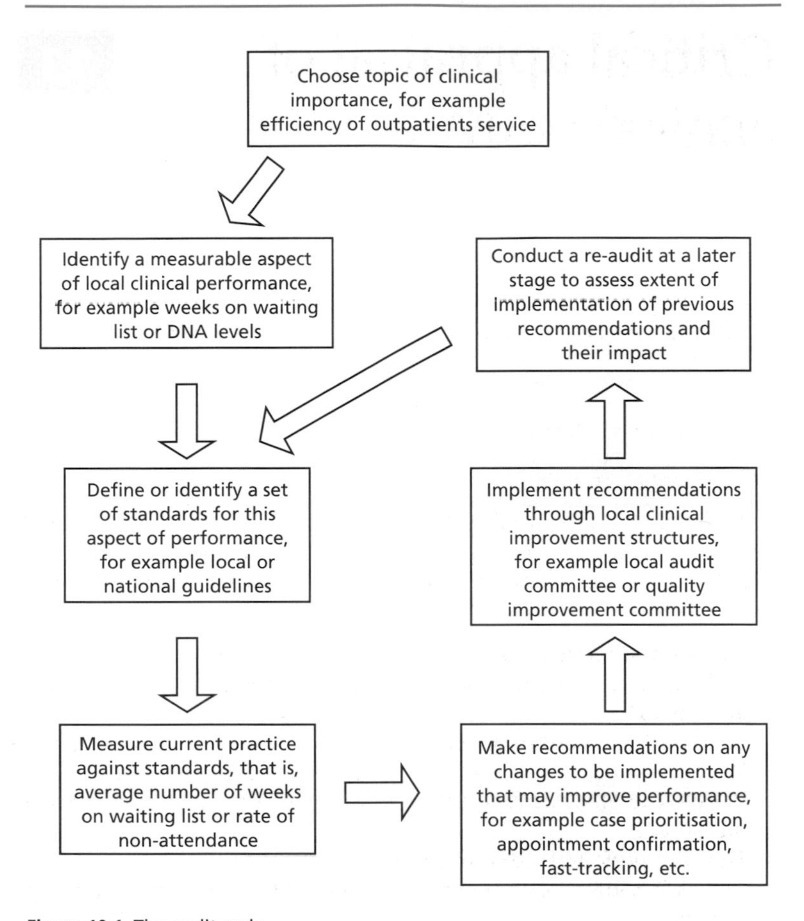

Figure 10.1 The audit cycle.

Critical appraisal of economic evaluations

11

It is not from the benevolence of the butcher, the brewer or the baker that we expect our dinner, but from their regard to their own self interest.

Adam Smith, *The Wealth of Nations* (1776)

Introduction

Economic evaluations present yet another type of evidence that may well feature in the critical review paper examination. The concepts described in economic evaluations can appear somewhat alien at first glance and medics may be disheartened by the unfamiliar economic jargon contained in these papers.

However, familiarization with the basic economic evaluation concepts will certainly show up these papers for what they really are – straightforward presentations of clinically important evidence! Candidates will also be reassured to know that economic evaluation reports are usually written in a format similar to the more familiar clinical papers such as randomized clinical trials, etc.

The material presented to clinicians by 'drug-reps' not only comprises data on comparative drug efficacies and side-effects but also includes separate data on comparative costs, derived from economic evaluations. Therefore, this is not as unfamiliar a territory as may be thought initially.

Economic evaluations are usually performed at the tail end of clinical trials and, here, costs and outcomes of concerned treatments are compared in order to determine how to best allocate often limited healthcare resources.

In this chapter, important concepts involved in making economic evaluations are discussed in detail, as well as the four main types of economic evaluations and their respective uses. A checklist for critically appraising economic evaluations is also included (p. 184).

Throughout this chapter, the terms 'costs' and 'outcomes' are used as below.

Sharon pays £10 (*cost*) for a hairdo! (*outcome*)

Costs and outcomes in health economics

Costs

'Costs' describes the total value of resources (money, time, energy, etc.) that are expended in the pursuance of an end.

Therefore, when 'Sharon' decides on a hairdo, the assigned cost in an economic evaluation would include the *direct* payment for service along with other costs, such as petrol costs or bus fares, etc. Also included will be *indirect* costs, such as the cost of her total time spent at the hairdressers, the cost of babysitting her one-year-old toddler and other costs associated with her loss of productivity during the outing.

'Opportunity costs' are defined as the cost of a decision in terms of the next best (*foregone*) alternative. This is in contrast to describing cost in terms of the direct value of purchase. Opportunity costs occur because humans have endless needs with limited resources to satisfy these needs. Choice, therefore, has to be made as to which needs are to be satisfied and with what priority.

EXAMPLE

Sharon is hungry and is also badly in need of a hairdo. Having only £10 to her name, she has two choices about how best to spend her limited resources. Coincidentally, both choices have equal monetary costs.

	Outcome	Cost	Opportunity cost
Choice 1	Meal	£10	Look horrible
Choice 2	Hairdo	£10	Hunger

In this scenario, Sharon may opt for Choice 1 because she rates the opportunity cost of a hairdo (*hunger!*) as being higher than that of a meal (*look horrible!*), even though both choices have equal direct costs. It is important, therefore, to consider the opportunity cost of any decision, as it may be greater in value than the direct cost of that decision.

Costs in healthcare

In a health-provision context, the 'direct' cost of Treatment Programme X would include all identifiable treatment costs along with other costs, such as project planning, building and premises, staff salaries, equipment, administration and so on. 'Indirect' costs would include patient-borne costs, such as absence from work and other duties during treatment period, loss of earnings and losses due to treatment side-effects, etc. Here, the 'opportunity' cost would be the value of other things that the resources used by Treatment Programme X would have been spent on otherwise, such as other treatment programmes.

Uncertainty

The concept of 'uncertainty' plays a large role in economic evaluations, and arises due to several factors. For instance, it is a generally accepted fact that benefits are deemed by people to have more value in the present than in the future, whereas current inconveniences are deemed worse than future ones.

Winning an exotic holiday to be taken later on this year would mean much more to most of us than if the said holiday were scheduled for 20 years from now. Finding true love now has more value than a guarantee of true love scheduled to occur in 10 years' time. Similarly, people would rather hand over the £5000 cost of a new car in 20 years' time than hand it in now.

This uncertainty about the future results from doubts about longevity of life, future health, future wealth, future inflation, future wars or famine, and even the apocalypse. Furthermore, most people apparently express a preference for the 'here and now', even when they are certain about future benefits ('pure time preference').

Time effects apart, uncertainty can also result from doubts about the degree of success that will be achieved by current ventures. These sources of uncertainty are the reasons and justification for the devaluation of benefits accruing from future events. This devaluation procedure is termed 'discounting' in economic evaluations.

Discounting

Discounting describes a process where present valuations are reduced according to a specified discount rate over time. This is in order to allow for the effects of uncertainty described above when calculating the costs and benefits of future events. Costs obtained after discounting are termed a 'net present value' (NPV) and represent the current worth of future events.

Discount rates used in economic evaluations do vary, depending on the country, the economy, the degree of uncertainty about future benefits, etc. In the UK, however, the Treasury discount rate for costs is set at 6% per annum.

EXAMPLE OF COSTS DISCOUNTING

A new radical treatment 'TXPDT' for arthritis has been estimated as costing £1,000,000 per patient annually. Total costs per patient over a 10-year period can be calculated after discounting, as follows:

Year	Annual cost of new treatment before discount	NPV @ 5% discount rate	NPV @ 10% discount rate
1	£1,000,000	£1,000,000	£1,000,000
2	£1,000,000	£907,029	£826,446
3	£1,000,000	£783,526	£620,921
4	£1,000,000	£644,609	£424,098
5	£1,000,000	£505,068	£263,331
6	£1,000,000	£376,889	£148,644
7	£1,000,000	£267,848	£76,278
8	£1,000,000	£181,290	£35,584
9	£1,000,000	£116,861	£15,091
10	£1,000,000	£71,743	£5818
Total costs	£10,000,000	£3,854,865	£2,416,211

NPV = net present value.

Ideally, all economic evaluations should present discounted costs (NPV) wherever applicable.

Outcomes

In economic evaluations, 'outcomes' are defined as the events that occur as a result of resource expenditure. Naturally, outcomes are widely varied, including anything from hairdos to organ transplants. The benefits derived from these outcomes are similarly endless in variety, including things such as satisfaction of biological drives, pleasure, comfort, convenience, health, longevity, etc.

Specific health outcomes can include things such as the lowering of blood cholesterol or blood pressure, early cancer detection, healthy births, stroke prevention, pain relief, restoration of normal mood, etc. Furthermore, some outcomes (early cancer detection) are generally costlier to society than others (lowering of blood pressure), whereas other outcomes (hip replacements) are viewed by society as more important than are others (liposuction).

In economic evaluations, the benefits conferred by various outcomes have to be quantified in such a way that comparisons can be made between competing or alternative outcomes. The trouble is how does one quantify outcomes?

Quantifying outcomes

Benefits derived from outcomes can either be quantified in terms of units identified as being 'natural' to the outcome being considered or in 'monetary' terms, or in terms of special economic units called 'utility'. (See the end of this chapter for specific details of how outcomes are quantified into monetary terms and utilities.)

Naturally occurring units

Outcomes can be quantified in terms of some identified naturally occurring unit that is logically and directly related to the benefits derived from them (Table 11.1). However, this may not be possible, with some outcomes (particularly in healthcare), whose benefits may be seen as being more vague and less tangible.

Table 11.1 Examples of naturally occurring units

Outcome	Naturally occurring units
Posted letter	Number of days to delivery
Battery	Battery life (hours)
Sports car	Top speed *or* 0–60 acceleration *or* miles per gallon
New centre forward (football)	Goals per season
Dialysis service	Patient life years saved
New anti-depressant	Depression days avoided
Pap smear programme	Number of cases detected

This method of quantifying outcomes is especially used in a type of economic evaluation called 'cost-effectiveness analysis'.

Monetary terms

Benefits can also be quantified in monetary terms. Here, health economists ascribe monetary values to the benefits derived from an outcome using some of the methods described in detail at the end of the chapter. The following are some examples:

- Successful treatment of heroin addiction may be valued as being worth £125,000 to society *vis-à-vis* increased productivity + less days off work + better parenting + less aggression + less crime, etc.
- Controlled childhood epilepsy may be valued as being worth £950,000 to society *vis-à-vis* less fits + better education + increased productivity for 60-years till retirement + less 999 calls, etc.
- Hip replacement may be valued as being worth £75,000 to society *vis-à-vis* pain relief + less disability + return to usual duties + fewer visits to GPs, etc.

Having quantified benefits into monetary terms, comparisons are then made between competing outcomes in economic evaluations. This method of quantifying outcomes is especially used in a type of economic evaluation called 'cost–benefit analysis'.

The main danger of this procedure is that there is huge potential for subjectivity and prejudice, depending on who is ascribing such monetary values. For example, an elderly lady may assign a higher value to hip replacements than would a younger adult, and the mother of a severely epileptic child may similarly view a cure for this condition as being worth much more than would a teenager.

Health economists or clinicians do not typically tend to be elderly ladies or mothers of epileptic children and thus there is always an element of subjectivity and bias.

Utility

The benefits derived from an outcome can similarly be described in terms of a special economic unit called 'utilities'. Utilities reflect the entirety of benefits derived from an outcome and are mainly used in a healthcare context.

Therefore, the utility ascribed to a hairdo may be given a subjective rating based on an array of derived benefits including things such as grooming, looking nice, time out from the home environment, gossip at the salon, information on hair-fashion, etc.

In a healthcare context, utilities tend to particularly reflect the 'quality of life' and 'longevity' aspects of healthcare benefits conferred onto patients. This is because, ultimately, all we want as people is to stay as healthy as possible for as long as possible.

'Quality of life' as a function of utility spans a scale of 0–1. Zero is ascribed to death and one to perfect health (maximum). Some health states are often ascribed scores less than zero, that is, worse than death. 'Longevity' as a function of utility is measured in terms of the number of years lived in a particular health state. Quality of life scores are usually combined with the number of years lived in that particular health state to produce an outcome measure called 'Quality adjusted life years' (QALYs). 1-QALY represents one year spent in full health. The example below illustrates how QALYs can be calculated for a particular health state.

	Ascribed quality of life	Expected life duration (years)	QALY
No treatment	0.3	2	0.6
After Treatment A	0.5	9	4.5
After Treatment B	0.8	5	4.0
After Treatment C	1	3	3

Having quantified benefits into utilities, comparisons are then made between competing outcomes in economic evaluations. From the above example, benefits derived from different treatments were quantified as utilities (QALYs), thus allowing for comparisons:

- Treatment A bestowed a gain of 3.9 QALYs.
- Treatment B bestowed a gain of 3.4 QALYs.
- Treatment C bestowed a gain of 2.4 QALYs.

This method of quantifying outcomes is especially used in a type of economic evaluation called 'cost–utility analyses'.

Discounting outcomes

Outcomes are discounted in economic evaluations in a similar way to costs. Although the example below illustrates how this is done, it is worth noting that compared to costs discounting, there is less consensus about how to discount outcomes. However, outcomes are usually discounted at a rate of 1.5% per annum.

EXAMPLE OF DISCOUNTING OUTCOMES

From clinical trials, a new treatment 'TXPDT' for arthritis shows promise of improving the 'quality of life' of sufferers by an average of 0.4 per year (0.4 QALYs). Total QALYs gained over a 10-year duration can be calculated after discounting, as follows (note: discount rate @ 1.5%):

Year	QALY gains pre-discount	Discounted QALY gains (NPV)
1	0.4	0.4
2	0.4	0.39
3	0.4	0.37
4	0.4	0.35
5	0.4	0.32
6	0.4	0.30
7	0.4	0.27
8	0.4	0.24
9	0.4	0.21
10	0.4	0.18
Total QALYs	4	2.62

So far, both the cost side and the outcome side of economic evaluations have been discussed. The next section examines the four types of economic evaluations and their indications. Decision-makers employ appropriate analyses in order to make decisions on the programmes that should have higher priority and the treatment methods that should be employed in achieving them.

Two prerequisites of any economic evaluation

- It must examine both the costs and outcomes of alternatives being compared.
- It must compare at least two such alternatives.

A study can only be described as an economic evaluation when these two criteria are fulfilled.

The four types of economic evaluations

- Cost-minimization analysis.
- Cost-effectiveness analysis.
- Cost–utility analysis.
- Cost–benefit analysis.

Cost-minimization analysis

This type of economic evaluation is performed in cases where competing outcomes are seen as being similar in nature (i.e. achieving similar goals) and, crucially, are shown to confer equal benefits, that is, are established as being equivalent. Since the outcomes under consideration confer equal benefits, comparisons can then be made on the basis of costs alone. However, the process of determining equivalence has to be justified, thorough and clearly stated in the economic evaluation.

EXAMPLE

Which would the cheaper way of reducing shoplifting crime in a shopping mall? Hire security guards from the 'Securis firm' or from the 'Securital firm'. Both firms have similar reputations and equal efficacy in reducing shoplifting crimes. The choice, therefore, surely comes down to costs.

Cost-minimization analysis

Firm	Efficacy (percentage crime reduction)	Annual costs
Securis	30%	£7500
Securital	30%	£7300

The above example illustrates how straightforward cost-minimization analyses can be. This lack of complexity is mainly because of the established equivalence of the outcomes being considered.

HEALTHCARE EXAMPLE

Which would be the cheaper way of treating depression? Prescribe an anti-depressant or prescribe a course of cognitive behavioural therapy. Both treatments have been shown in randomized trials as having equal efficacies in the reduction of depressive symptoms. A cost-minimization analysis would be appropriate here.

Cost-minimization analysis in healthcare

Outcome	Efficacy	Total costs for 6 months
Anti-depressant treatment	66% Restoration of normal mood at 6 months	£620
Cognitive behavioural therapy	66% Restoration of normal mood at 6 months	£750

Table 11.2 Examples of naturally occurring units

Competing outcomes	Commonly shared outcome measure	Comparison measure
Toothpaste versus dental floss	Caries avoided yearly	Cost per caries avoided
Drive to work versus train to work	Days late avoided yearly	Cost per day late avoided
Anti-depressants versus CBT	Depression days avoided	Cost per depression day avoided
Dialysis versus transplant	Life year saved	Cost per life year saved

CBT = cognitive behavioural therapy.

Cost-effectiveness analysis

This type of economic evaluation is performed in cases where competing outcomes are seen as being similar in nature (i.e. achieving similar goals) but are deemed to be non-equivalent in the magnitude or quality of benefits they confer (i.e. unequal benefits).

In other words, when outcomes are seen as achieving similar effects but differ regarding the size of those effects, a choice can be made between these outcomes, based on an identified commonly shared outcome measure such as the 'naturally occurring units' described earlier (p. 172). The cost per unit of commonly shared outcome measure can be worked out in order to make comparisons as shown in Table 11.2.

EXAMPLE

What is the best way of reducing shoplifting crime in a shopping mall? Install CCTV or hire a firm of security guards? The identified outcome measure for comparison in this instance could be a 'percentage crime reduction' measure or even a 'number of annual arrests' measure.

Cost-effectiveness analysis

	Annual cost	Percentage crime reduction	Annual arrests	Cost per 1% reduction	Cost per arrest
CCTV	£20,000	10% reduction	60	£2000	£333
Security guards	£55,000	16% reduction	142	£3438	£387

Clearly, CCTV costs £1438 less per 1% reduction or £54 less per arrest than the security guards and therefore is more cost-effective.

Some purchasers, however, may view the extra benefits provided by the security guard option with keen interest despite the higher cost and lower cost-effectiveness. In order to elucidate matters further, an incremental cost-effectiveness calculation may have to be made.

INCREMENTAL COST-EFFECTIVENESS (COST PER SINGLE EXTRA UNIT OF BENEFIT)

Whenever one alternative costs more and also provides more benefits than another alternative (as with the example above), a clearer sense of cost-effectiveness can be obtained by calculating an incremental cost-effectiveness ratio. This ratio can be defined as the cost per single extra unit of benefit and is obtained by dividing the incremental (extra) costs by the incremental (*extra*) benefits.

In the above example, an incremental cost-effectiveness calculation would shed light on the exact cost per unit of extra benefit provided by the security guard option as shown below.

Incremental cost-effectiveness of the security guard option

	Incremental cost	Incremental percentage crime reduction	Cost per extra 1% reduction	Incremental arrests	Cost per extra arrest
Security guards	£35,000	6% reduction	£5833	82	£427

From the above data, the incremental benefits (extra 6% reduction or extra 82 arrests) conferred by the security guards option came at an extra cost of £35,000. Specifically, £5833 for every extra 1% crime reduction over the 10% figure obtained with CCTV or £427 for every additional arrest beyond the 60 arrests figure for CCTV. Whether this incremental cost is justified or not would be a matter of opinion.

This is the main strength of using incremental cost-effectiveness. It provides deeper insights into costs by clarifying the exact cost of extra benefits. Incremental cost–utility and incremental cost–benefit measures are also used in those respective types of economic analyses.

HEALTHCARE EXAMPLE

What is the most cost-effective way of treating renal failure? Invest in a dialysis unit or a renal transplant unit. The identifiable common outcome measure here could be a 'life year saved' measure. The table below illustrates a preliminary cost-effectiveness analysis performed before discounting.

Cost-effectiveness analysis in healthcare			
	Lives saved annually	Annual costs	Cost per life year saved
Dialysis	150	£1,000,000	£6667
Transplant	240	£2,500,000	£10,417

Clearly, a dialysis programme appears more cost-effective than a transplant programme as it costs £6667 per life year saved compared with £10,417 with a transplant programme, a difference of £3750.

However, conducting an incremental cost-effectiveness analysis, as shown below, reveals a £16,667 cost per extra life saved in a transplant programme over and above the 150 lives saved in a dialysis programme. Whether the additional benefit is worth the incremental cost would be a matter of judgement for the purchasers.

Incremental cost-effectiveness			
	Extra lives saved annually	Extra annual costs	Cost per extra life year saved
Transplant	90	£1,500,000	£16,667

The table below illustrates a full-blown cost-effectiveness analysis over a projected 20-year period, with discount rates of 5% and 1.5% used for costs and outcomes, respectively.

Year	Dialysis discounted		Transplant discounted	
	Lives saved annually (NPV)	Annual costs (NPV)	Lives saved annually (NPV)	Annual costs (NPV)
1	150	£1,000,000	240	£2,500,000
2	146	£907,029	233	£2,267,574
3	139	£783,526	223	£1,958,815
4	131	£644,609	210	£1,611,522
5	122	£505,068	195	£1,262,670
6	111	£376,889	178	£942,224
7	100	£267,848	161	£669,621
8	89	£181,290	143	£453,226
9	78	£116,861	125	£292,153
10	67	£71,743	107	£179,357
11	57	£41,946	91	£104,866
12	48	£23,357	76	£58,393
13	39	£12,387	63	£30,967
14	32	£6256	51	£15,641
15	26	£3009	41	£7523
16	20	£1379	32	£3447

Year	Dialysis discounted		Transplant discounted	
	Lives saved annually (NPV)	Annual costs (NPV)	Lives saved annually (NPV)	Annual costs (NPV)
17	16	£601	25	£1504
18	12	£250	19	£625
19	9	£99	14	£247
20	7	£37	11	£93
Total	1398	£4,944,187 Cost per life saved = £3537	2237	£12,360,468 Cost per life saved = £5526

Cost–utility analysis

As opposed to naturally occurring units or monetary units, cost–utility analyses describe benefits in terms of utilities. The most commonly used type of utility is the 'quality adjusted life year' (QALY) that captures both the quality and duration elements of derived benefits.

QALYs are obtained by combining quality values of health states with the number of years spent in such states. As we have already seen, 1-QALY is equivalent to one-year lived in full health. (See the end of this chapter for specific details of how we arrive at quality values.)

Because 'quality-of-life' measures are applicable across most aspects of healthcare, utilities are therefore a versatile method of making comparisons between even the most varied of health outcomes. This is a main strength of cost–utility analyses and thus they are applicable whenever the health outcomes being compared are different in nature (*different goals*), therefore producing completely different types of health benefits.

EXAMPLE

On which of these two alternatives should our friend Sharon spend her £1000 savings?

- A £900 facelift that will last for eight years and improve her quality of life from 0.5 to 0.9 (self-esteem confidence, etc.), or
- A £700 car that will last for 10 years and improve her quality of life from 0.5 to 0.8 (improvement of social isolation, convenience, etc.).

Cost–utility analysis					
Outcome	Cost	Quality gained	Duration (years)	QALYs	Cost per QALY
Facelift	£900	0.4	8	3.2	£281
Car	£700	0.3	10	3	£233

(Note: it must be said, that for the sake of clarity, deliberately low values have been used in the 'quality gained' column. Lack of a car or the need for a facelift would never result in such low quality of life scores in real life!)

Therefore Sharon can be advised that she would be spending £48 more per QALY, if she decides on a facelift instead of a car. In reality, cost–utility analyses are reserved only for health economics because the concept of quality of life is inextricably linked with health and health states.

HEALTHCARE EXAMPLE

A hospital manager with a limited budget is in two minds:

- Fund a £900 hip replacement operation on a severely arthritic 68-year-old woman, which would improve her quality of life from 0.5 to 0.9 for a duration of 10 years.
- Fund a £2500 behavioural programme for a seven-year-old autistic boy, which would improve his quality of life from 0.3 to 0.5 for a duration of 60 years.

Cost–utility analysis in healthcare

Outcome	Cost	Quality gained	Duration (years)	QALYs	Cost per QALY
Hip replacement	£900	0.4	10	4	£225
Behavioural programme	£2500	0.2	60	12	£208

As demonstrated in this example, despite much higher costs, the behavioural programme appears to be a more prudent expenditure than the hip replacement operation because of a lower cost per QALY figure.

Thankfully with these real-life quandaries, other principles come into play when resource allocation decisions are made. These include societal values, morals, urgency of need, political pressures, physical pain, etc.

COST–UTILITY IN ACTION

Below are some cost–utility analysis exercises to have some fun with. Work out the cost per QALY for each scenario and prioritize each case in order of merit, initially using QALYs alone and then using your own clinical judgement. What other principles may have informed your judgement apart from economic? How much different from a straight 'cost per QALY' rating is your priority listing? Such are the weaknesses of cost–utility analyses.

1 Mr Smith, a 77-year-old retired policeman, lives with his loving wife and has just been diagnosed with colon cancer. He is in need of urgent life-saving surgery, which would add three years to his life, albeit in a state of health of 0.6, due to problems arising from radiotherapy, bowel surgery and a colostomy, etc. Cost of surgery is £5600.
2 Ms Potter, a 37-year-old unemployed mother of three, has pelvic pain due to severe endriometriosis. Her gynaecologist has advised a radical hysterectomy which would improve her quality of life from 0.6 to 0.9 for another 20 years, albeit on hormone replacement therapy. Cost of surgery is £4200.
3 Mr Hutchinson, a 43-year-old married father of two, has intractable heart failure following a recent myocardial infarction and will die without surgery. With surgery he will live for another 10 years in a health state of 0.7. Cost of surgery is £5800.
4 Ms Mulligan, a 42-year-old lady, has been trying unsuccessfully for a baby with her long-term partner for five years and wants IVF treatment. It is felt that a baby would improve her quality of life from 0.9 to 1 for the remaining 30 years of her life. Cost of treatment is £3500.
5 Miss Cook, a 23-year-old attractive air hostess, has disfiguring facial scarring from a violent rape incident that occurred on an overnight stop in a foreign country. Despite making progress in counselling, her therapist feels strongly that cosmetic surgery will improve her health state by a factor of 0.4. She will live to 89 years of age. Cost of surgery is £2900.
6 Mr Jones, a 40-year-old NHS consultant, has a slipped disk and chronic back pain. He has been on sick leave for six months and is in need of a laminectomy, which would improve his quality of life from 0.4 to 0.8 and facilitate his return to work. He is expected to live for another 35 years. Cost of surgery is £2400.
7 Karen is a 17-year-old girl with morbid obesity. Her doctors are in agreement that, as a last resort, gastric stapling may help reduce her weight and, therefore, her risk of mortality. Her quality of life is expected to improve by a factor of 0.2 and she may live for another 50 years with a health state of 1. Cost of surgery is £2500.
8 Lucy, formerly known as Joshua, is an award-winning 27-year-old school teacher. She wants facial electrolysis to complete her gender reassignment programme. It is felt that her current beard reduces her quality of life by 0.1 and affects her confidence, particularly at

school. She will live for another 50 years with a health state of 1. Cost of surgery is £1300.

9 Mr Stevens is a 22-year-old man on a five-year prison sentence for aggravated burglary. He requires an operation to remove nasal polyps, which cause him severe headaches amongst other problems. His quality of life is expected to improve from 0.8 to 1 after the operation. Surgeons can only guarantee non-recurrence for the first five years after the operation. Cost of surgery is £2600.

10 Ben, a two-year-old boy with Down's syndrome and a large ventricular septal defect, is expected to live for another year unless he has a heart transplant. With a transplant he will live for another 10 years with his health state improved from 0.2 to 0.8. Cost of surgery is £8800.

Cost–benefit analysis

In cost–benefit analyses, all benefits derived from an outcome are assigned a monetary value, as opposed to utilities or naturally occurring units. The monetary value of these benefits are then combined with respective costs, forming a 'benefit–cost ratio'.

If having a hairdo costs a total of £30 (including all the indirect costs described earlier) and all the benefits derived from that activity were evaluated as being worth £150, the 'benefit–cost ratio' would be five (150/30).

Because benefits of all kinds can be theoretically assigned a monetary value, comparisons can be made between widely dissimilar outcomes in cost–benefit analyses. This versatility is a main advantage, as with cost–utility analyses.

There are, however, questions about the validity of assigning monetary values to things such as pain relief, restoration of normal mood, saving a life, etc. This is a major flaw of cost–benefit analyses that makes them so controversial.

EXAMPLE

Again, our hospital manager with a limited budget is in two minds about which of the two treatment interventions to pursue:

- Fund a £900 hip replacement operation on a severely arthritic 68-year-old woman, which would improve her quality of life for a duration of 10 years. Cured arthritis of a single hip joint is valued as providing £350,000 worth of benefits over the 10 years.

- Fund a £2500 behavioural programme for a seven-year-old autistic boy, which would improve his quality of life for a duration of 60 years. The benefits conferred by such a programme are valued as being worth £1,250,000 over the 60-year period.

Cost–benefit analysis of hip replacement and behavioural programme

Outcome	Cost	Worth of benefits	Benefit–cost ratio
Hip replacement	£900	£350,000	389
Behavioural programme	£2500	£1,250,000	500

From the information above, the hospital manager may decide that the behavioural programme offers better value for money because of its greater benefit–cost ratio, that is, more benefits per unit cost.

By indicating an order in which projects might be commissioned, cost–benefit analyses are particularly useful as a rough guide to policy-makers when making decisions about resource allocation. In such scenarios, societal projects with higher benefit–cost ratios would have priority over those with lower ratios.

Again, other factors do thankfully come into play when resource allocation decisions are made.

Critical appraisal of economic evaluations – a checklist

Critical appraisal of economic evaluations should always begin with an assessment of the primary economic question under consideration. Does the primary question address a clinically important issue or area of practice? (Figure 11.1).

Listed below are the main considerations when assessing the strengths and weaknesses of economic evaluations (see Table 11.3 as well).

- Is the primary economic question clearly stated and does it address a clinically important issue?
- Is the pre-evaluation stance of the authors clearly stated?
- Is there a clear statement of the aims and objectives of the evaluation?
- Is the choice of economic evaluation appropriate in light of the three previous considerations?
- Are the outcomes being considered clearly stated?
- Is the rationale for choosing the comparison outcomes justified in light of current clinical practice?

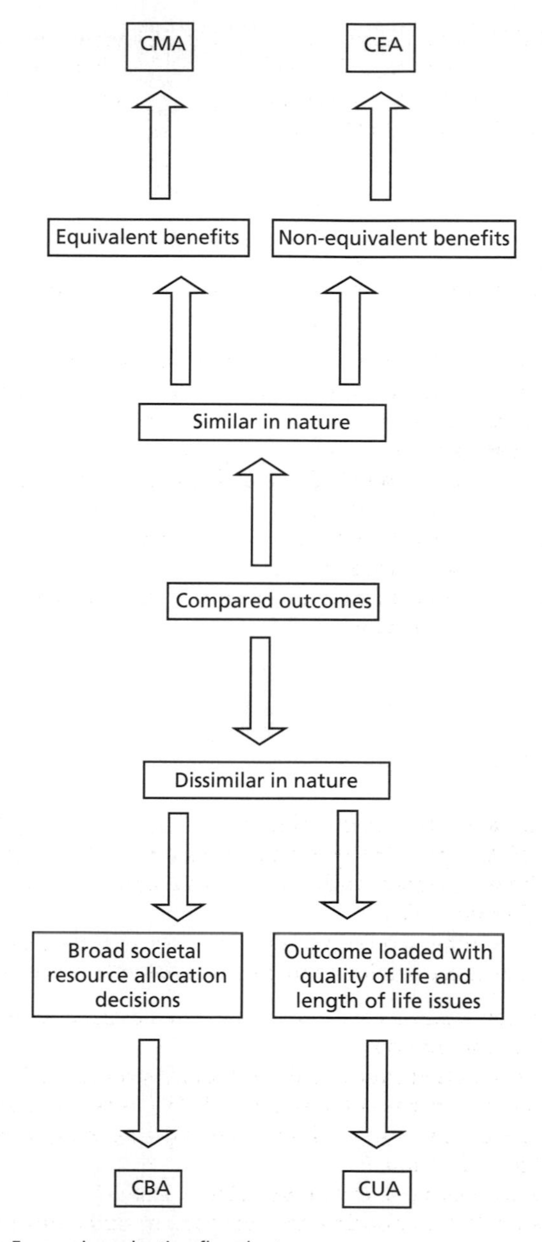

Figure 11.1 Economic evaluation flowchart.

Table 11.3 Strengths and weaknesses of the respective economic analyses

	Cost-minimization	Cost-effectiveness	Cost–utility	Cost–benefit
Simplicity	Simple	Moderately simple	Complex	Complex
Relationship of chosen outcome measure to benefits	Directly relevant	Directly relevant	Ascribed (utility)	Ascribed (monetary)
Versatility	One-dimensional (similar outcomes and equal benefit)	One-dimensional (similar outcomes and unequal benefits)	Multi-dimensional (dissimilar outcomes and benefits)	Multi-dimensional (dissimilar outcomes and benefits)
Range of use in healthcare	Narrow	Limited	Extensive	Extensive
Uses outside healthcare	Yes	Yes	Truly meaningful only in a health context	Yes
Outcome quantification	Already established	Internally derived	? Validity of methodology	? Validity of methodology
Degree of subjectivity	Low	Low–moderate	High	High
Prejudice factor (ageist, sexist, etc.)	Low	Low	High	High

- Are the chosen outcome measures clearly stated and do these reasonably capture the expected benefits from outcomes?
- Are the sources of data on efficacy of the outcomes stated and, if so, are these sources credible? If CMA, how was equivalence established?
- Are the methods of outcome quantification clearly stated and justified?
- Are all relevant benefits included when quantifying outcomes?
- Are future benefits discounted?
- Is the chosen discount rate stated and justified?
- Do the authors clearly show how the costs for compared outcomes were estimated?
- Are all relevant costs included and, if not, was this stated and justified?
- Are the costs estimates reasonable?
- Are costs discounted? Is the chosen discount rate stated and justified?
- Is an incremental analysis performed?
- Is a sensitivity analysis performed and how is this justified? (See end of chapter.)
- Are the conclusions from the economic analysis stated?

Non-essential information

Specific methods used in outcome measurement

A large number of people are surveyed about the following.

WILLINGNESS TO PAY

How much are people willing to pay in order to achieve perfect health from a given condition, for example gallstones. This would indicate the monetary cost of a cure of gallstones.

CATEGORY RATING

To rate on a visual analogue scale between death >- - - - - - - - - - < perfect health where they think a described disease state should be, for example, stroke hemiplegia. This would indicate the quality of life in that disease state. May be worse than death in some health states!

STANDARD GAMBLE

What risks of death are people willing to accept in an attempt to get perfect health from a described disease state. This would indicate the value of life in that illness state.

TIME TRADE-OFF

How many of their remaining years in a disease state they would trade-off for a chance at perfect health. This would indicate the value of life in that disease state.

Sensitivity analysis

Economic evaluations are about comparing the costs and benefits of alternative outcomes. As evident thus far, quantifying costs and benefits involves making several estimations based on various assumptions about the costs and benefits. Estimates always carry a degree of uncertainty and in economic analyses these uncertainties can in turn affect the validity of results.

Sensitivity analyses are, therefore, performed in order to increase the validity of economic analysis results. In this procedure, values of estimated parameters are repeatedly tinkered with so as to test the consistency of the results over a range of assumptions.

For example, the estimated costs of the transplant and dialysis units can be methodically varied in order to assess any effects on cost-effectiveness figures. The benefit estimates on the number of lives saved can also be similarly varied. The more thorough the sensitivity analysis, the more robust the result findings of an economic evaluation are deemed to be.

Specific methods used in sensitivity analyses

The estimates for which a sensitivity analysis is needed are first identified along with a plausible range of values over which they are thought to vary. One of the following ways of conducting a sensitivity analysis is then applied to data.

- Simple one-way sensitivity analysis – altering the value of one parameter at a time.
- Simple multi-way sensitivity analysis – altering the values of two or more sets of parameters simultaneously.

ANALYSIS OF EXTREMES

Estimates of all identified parameters are set to values at the extremes of their respective ranges in such a way as to model a best-case scenario or a worst-case scenario.

EXAMPLE

Best dialysis scenario or worst dialysis scenario:

	Lives saved annually	Annual costs	Lives saved annually	Annual costs
Dialysis	Highest plausible estimate	Lowest plausible estimate	Lowest plausible estimate	Highest plausible estimate
Transplant	Lowest plausible estimate	Highest plausible estimate	Highest plausible estimate	Lowest plausible estimate

THRESHOLD SENSITIVITY ANALYSIS

Estimates can be varied in such a way as to find the critical point at which a reversal of conclusions occurs. This set of threshold values can then be examined regarding their closeness to believed realistic values.

Critical appraisal of qualitative studies

12

What is qualitative research?

In a healthcare setting, qualitative research can be thought of as 'the systematic exploration of a research question using interpretative, naturalistic and holistic methodologies'.

What does this mean?

In contrast to quantitative studies, where emphasis is placed on the measured quantities of observed phenomena, qualitative methodologies are geared towards the exploration of less tangible and less easily measured phenomena such as the meanings, attitudes, beliefs or behaviours people may have in relation to a relevant property. In other words, a sort of 'behind the scenes' humanistic focus and approach to answering a medical research question.

A qualitative researcher seeks to explore the human experiential interpretation of any observed phenomena. This is called the 'interpretative' element of qualitative research and it enables researchers to gain a better understanding of the underlying processes that may influence the data observations in a study.

Another distinction between qualitative and quantitative research is that with qualitative methods, the examination of a research question takes place in the natural setting where the concerned subject matter normally exists. This 'naturalistic' element of qualitative research ensures that the natural state of the measured property is not disturbed. Quantitative methods, such as randomised clinical trials on the other hand, often involve the application of artificial experimental conditions to the area of interest as a pre-requisite to taking 'objective' measurements of the concerned property.

Qualitative research principles also encourage the exploration of a research question multi-dimensionally, exhaustively and in its entirety, i.e. a 'holistic' approach that takes into account any relevant tangential, or satellite issues arising from the research. This is why a fair degree of flexibility and creativity is needed in qualitative methodology to collect all relevant data.

Background

Qualitative and quantitative research methods derive their principles from two opposing schools of thought in social anthropology, naturalism and positivism, respectively (Figure 12.1).

Types of qualitative methodologies

There are different methodological approaches in qualitative research. When conducting a qualitative project, the researcher needs to select the methodology they feel will be most suitable to the nature of the research question at hand.

Grounded theory

Grounded theory, as described by Glaser and Strauss in 1967, is by far the most commonly encountered and widely used qualitative methodology. Although different researchers have different interpretations of the original doctrine, the core principles of grounded theory can be summarized as below.

Naturalism

- Only the internal subjective world exists
- Reality is a subjective entity
- The *truth* exists in subjective reality
- There are many realities, i.e., reality is a subjective construct

Qualitative research principles

- Naturalistic
- Interpretative
- Holistic
- Inductive, i.e., theory generation (observation → theory)
- 'TORCH LIGHT' approach

Positivism

- A real external world exists out there
- Reality is an objective entity
- The *truth* exists in objective reality
- Only one objective reality

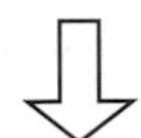

Quantitative research principles

- Experimental
- Quantifying
- Standardized
- Deterministic, i.e., theory testing (theory → observation)
- 'TAPE MEASURE' approach

Figure 12.1 Naturalism and positivism.

When embarking on a qualitative project, researchers should ideally not harbour any 'a priori hypotheses' or tendencies on the concerned subject matter i.e., before making their observations. Therefore, any themes generated should ideally be generated purely from data observations. This principle is termed 'emergence' in grounded theory.

In other words, there is no concept of a null or alternative hypothesis in the grounded theory approach to qualitative research. All emergent theories from a qualitative project should ideally be 'grounded' in the reality of the obtained data. The grounded theory methodology can also be described as being 'inductive' in that researchers are encouraged to explore any new or unforeseen issues that may arise during the qualitative research process. This encouraged exploration often results in tangential pursuits in a qualitative study but ensures that researchers get a full picture of the property being investigated.

Another principle of grounded theory is that when conducting a qualitative research project, analysis of data begins right from the stage of data collection i.e. data collection and data analysis are carried out *simultaneously*. This interesting feature facilitates the inductive process and the process of emergence in qualitative research. As can be expected, however, the degree to which qualitative researchers adhere to this principle varies on a continuum that ranges from that of purism to pragmatism. Other core principles of grounded theory such as 'theoretical sampling' and the 'constant-comparative method' of analysis are discussed in the relevant sections below.

Other qualitative methodologies – not essential

- Interpretative phenomenological analysis (IPA) approach.
- Discourse analysis approach.
- Content analysis approach.
- Narrative analysis approach.
- Ethnographic analysis approach.

See qualitative research text for details.

(Note: For the remainder of this chapter, qualitative research principles will be explored only from the grounded theory perspective.)

When are qualitative methods appropriate?

Qualitative research methods are useful for when evaluating clinical research questions in a new field of study, often as a prelude to conducting quantitative studies on a subject matter. Also, certain complex, intangible, abstract or salient clinical issues can be explored better and with more depth only by using qualitative methods. This is because qualitative methods are better geared to exploring the human experiences, feelings, attitudes, and behaviour that underlie the observed phenomena of interest in a subject area.

Qualitative research methods are also useful for situations when quantitative methods have been frustrated. In such instances, such as where quantitative methods have produced unexplainable or contradictory results, further exploration of data can be done with qualitative methods so as to generate explanatory theories. This is a very common practice.

In essence, *qualitative methods reach the parts of a subject matter that other methods cannot reach.*

Listed below are the kinds of research questions that can be answered with qualitative research methods.

Clinical questions with a 'contextual focus' aim to *identify* and *describe*:

- What are the experiences of relatives visiting patients in this hospital?
- What are the attitudes of young people on safe sex?
- What is the ethnic-minority community perception of psychotherapy?

Clinical questions with a 'diagnostic focus' aim to find *explanations*:

- Why has there been a rise in the number of complaints made by visitors to this hospital?
- Why has there been a poor response from young people to the safe sex programme?
- Why do ethnic-minority patients rarely receive psychotherapy?

Clinical questions with an 'evaluative focus' aim to assess *effectiveness*:

- Are visitors to this hospital satisfied with the new car parking system?
- Is the safe sex programme meeting the needs of young people?
- Are there more than usual access barriers to psychotherapy for ethnic-minority patients?

Clinical questions with a 'strategic focus' aim to improve:

- How do people think vehicle congestion can be further improved during visiting hours?
- How do young people think safe sex programmes can be better implemented?
- How can access to psychotherapy be made easier for ethnic-minority patients?

Qualitative data collection methods

Structured interviews

In these interviews, subjects are given a set of structured questions either by questionnaire or by a trained interviewer who administers the questions in a standardized format.

Structured questions are closed questions that have limited response choices, thereby restricting the depth and variety of responses that can be obtained from the interviewees. This is a major disadvantage of structured interviews because respondents are forced into the provided response sets or categories. Responders may feel that they had no room to express their opinions accurately.

The advantages of structured interviews are that they can be delivered to a large number of people over a relatively short time period at reduced costs. They are also infinitely easier to analyze.

Semi-structured interviews

These interviews adhere to an overall loose structure. Major questions are organized in such a way as to constitute the spine or agenda of the interview. These major questions may then branch out to a more open type of questioning where interviewees are allowed to offer more detailed responses.

By drawing on the advantages of the two types of interviews, semi-structured interviews are able to generate more individualized and more accurate data than structured interviews whilst still maintaining an overall sense of structure that can be so invaluable even when analyzing qualitative data.

In-depth interviews

Here, issues are covered in great detail and questions are asked in an open-ended format. This type of interview has no fixed pre-set agenda and respondents are allowed to lead the interview and to give their full responses. It is encouraged that ongoing questioning during an in-depth interview is based on the responses just obtained from the interviewee in order that the interviewer be able to explore the subject matter comprehensively. This is called 'probing' in an in-depth interview.

Some loose degree of structure does exist with in-depth interviews, in that the interviewer may have a listed reminder of issues or areas to be covered during the interview. These are called 'topic guides'. Newly emergent issues from an interview may be added to the topic guides for subsequent interviews, i.e., an 'inductive' process.

In-depth interviews can last for two hours or more and they are the mainstay or gold standard of data collection methods in qualitative research. In-depth interviews are usually recorded and transcribed into text for further analysis when they are examined along with contemporaneous notes.

Focus groups

Focus groups classically comprise 8–12 people who have been deliberately brought together to discuss a commonly shared issue. One or two facilitators conduct the group by non-directive questioning, observation, clarification, etc. Focus group sessions are usually recorded on tape and transcribed into text for analysis.

Focus groups can provide a wide breadth of opinion on a subject matter in a relatively short space of time. Therefore, qualitative researchers at the start of a project often use focus groups to rapidly generate a wide variety of issues on the subject of interest.

The disadvantages of focus groups are mostly to do with the dynamics that occur in any kind of group. More vocal people in a group tend to dominate discussion whilst the opinions of the more reluctant participants often get stifled. Group dynamics are very powerful indeed and can alter the opinions of all group members towards a central or even extreme consensus opinion, thereby affecting the very validity of the data obtained in such focus groups.

Because groups can be very *busy*, the information obtained from focus groups is often voluminous but lacking in real depth. This makes the transcription of a record of a focus group a very onerous task.

Observational methods

Observational methods are best suited for qualitative research questions that are loaded with behavioural or procedural issues. Rather than just record the likely inaccurate responses from people about their behaviours, observational methods allow qualitative researchers to assess human behaviours and interactions first-hand, along with the impact these behaviours may have on the subject of interest.

The major limitation of observational methods is that the very presence of an observer can alter people's behaviour. The magnitude of this alteration and its impact on the property of interest can be almost impossible to determine. To overcome this problem, under appropriate circumstances, some qualitative researchers may justifiably embark on covert observational methods.

Observational methods (overt and covert) are frequently used in the area of health management to identify areas of weakness and possible strategies for healthcare improvement. Yes … you may be under observation as we speak … be afraid, be very afraid!

Sampling in qualitative research

The process of selecting subjects in qualitative research involves a very different process from that used in quantitative studies. In grounded theory based qualitative research, subjects are strategically selected based on their identified potential for providing information that can extend or test pre-existing understanding on a subject matter. In other words, selection of subjects is strategic, active, systematic and deliberate, and emphasis is placed on the gathering of as much information as possible with which to examine current theoretical constructs on a subject matter.

This manner of selection is called 'theoretical sampling'. Therefore, when faced with a research question, a qualitative researcher strategically selects information-rich cases (as opposed to random sampling in quantitative studies).

Different kinds of theoretical sampling

Convenience sampling

Sampling is conducted by selecting those who are readily accessible or available and to whom the research question applies. For example, in a qualitative study aiming to explore the experiences of doctors when in a reversed role of being patients themselves, convenience sampling may be carried out by simply recruiting all doctors who present as patients to a hospital department over a given time period.

Quota sampling

Sampling is conducted by allocating quotas to a set of criteria that are identified as being important to the research question. Cases are then selected in order to fulfil these. Going with the doctor role-reversal example, important criteria for selecting participant doctors may include male:female ratio, levels of medical experience, doctors from different specialities etc.

Typical case sampling

Sampling is conducted by deliberately selecting only those cases that have been identified as possessing all the characteristics of a typical case in relation to the relevant subject area.

Maximum variation sampling

Sampling is conducted by deliberately selecting cases that have the most divergent or dissimilar characteristics. This is usually done in order to generate as many diverse views as possible on the research question, or in order to test the emerging trends occurring during a study. In grounded theory, the practice of sampling dissimilar cases is also an important aspect of ascertaining validity of qualitative data. See later section.

Snowball sampling

Sampling is conducted based on obtaining information about potential contacts from key subject(s). Key subjects can be professionals who work in the relevant subject area e.g. sex-workers or drug counsellors or the actual potential participants themselves e.g. prostitutes or heroin addicts. This sampling strategy can 'snowball' rapidly as every identified subject becomes a potential source of more contacts who are then traced, consented, recruited and fleeced for more information on contacts. Snowball sampling is most helpful when conducting research amongst these kinds of groups that are otherwise inaccessible.

Because data analysis proceeds concurrently with data collection in qualitative research, sampling strategies can and should be regularly revised and modified as necessary during the research process.

Sample size in qualitative research

In qualitative research, the sample size of a study is chiefly determined by practical constraints such as time and resources by the phenomenon of 'saturation'. Saturation in a qualitative study occurs whenever it can be reasonably concluded that the recruitment of additional cases no longer provide additional information or insights to the level of understanding achieved with the subject area.

Analysis of qualitative data

As an inductive process, qualitative data analysis is a continuous process that begins right from the stage of data collection and carries on throughout the research process. On the whole, data analysis involves a systematic approach, where the researcher seeks to identify any major recurrent themes and subthemes in the data.

Qualitative data usually exists in a transcribed textual format, which can be highly voluminous considering the huge amount of information that can be collected from just a single in-depth interview! However, by a process of sorting, coding, cutting and pasting, data are organized into several labelled categories and subcategories based on the identified themes and subthemes – this is called a 'thematic framework'.

(Note: This process of data coding can be facilitated by a number of available software packages.)

Having organized qualitative data into a thematic framework,themes are examined and charted in order to record and theorise on any emergent trends, associations or causal relationships. This method of analyzing qualitative data in grounded theory qualitative research is known as the 'constant comparative method'.

The critical appraisal of qualitative studies asks:

- Is the study design methodologically sound?
- What do the results show?
- How do the results affect the care of my patients?

Is the study design methodologically sound?

The following are the main considerations when assessing the validity of qualitative research studies, i.e., the strengths and weaknesses of qualitative designs.

Does the study address an important clinical issue?

As with any type of study, the initial consideration when appraising a qualitative study is of the primary research question being addressed by the researchers. An assessment of the importance of the research question being addressed in a qualitative study should be made. Generally, important qualitative studies are those that increase the depth of understanding of major clinical issues or those that focus on salient or overlooked clinical areas that may have appreciable quality of life implications.

Was a qualitative design appropriate in answering the research question?

A determination needs to be made as to whether qualitative methods were appropriate for examining the research question. Qualitative methods are best suited for research questions where people's attitudes, beliefs or behaviour regarding a clinical issue need to be explored. Qualitative methods are also indicated in scenarios where quantitative methods are not expected to offer much insight into the subject of interest.

For example, the research question: 'What are the attitudes of teenage mothers towards breastfeeding?' may be better approached with a qualitative design, whereas the question: 'Do teenage mothers breastfeed for a shorter duration compared with older mothers?' may be better answered with a quantitative design.

Are the aims of the study clearly defined?

Admittedly, qualitative aims are generally more intricate and broader in scope than those of quantitative studies. Nevertheless, the overall aims of a qualitative study need to be clearly and concisely described in the study report. Wherever applicable, an account should also be given of any broadening of aims that may have occurred during the study as part of the *inductive* ethos of qualitative methodology.

How were the cases selected?

The selection methods used in a qualitative study should be clearly described and justified by the authors. A description of the subjects involved in a qualitative study should also be given so that the reader is able to pass judgements on the validity of the obtained data. The report should show how the selection process was systematic as well as the assumptions that made researchers believe that subjects would be rich information sources.

Was the process of method of data collection adequately described?

The entire process of data collection in a qualitative study should be described in adequate detail when presenting result findings. Issues such as the settings where interviews or focus groups were held, types of questioning used, use of questionnaires, observational methods and even a topic guide can all affect the very nature of data collected and should be described in detail. An adequate description allows readers to make comparisons with their own experiences.

Are the chosen methods of data collection justified?

The chosen data collection methods should be justified in the report of a qualitative study. For example, researchers may choose to adopt a semi-structured interview format instead of an in-depth interview format in a qualitative study when addressing a finite research question with limited scope. Transparency in reporting a qualitative study is crucial because it enables the reader to pass better judgements on the merits of the study design and any information gathered.

Is the process of data analysis adequately described?

As mentioned earlier (p. 191), qualitative data analysis should begin at the stage of data collection with researchers continuously trying to make sense of collected data, identifying and theorising about any recurring themes and inductively exploring any new angles.

Authors should offer sufficient explanations on the reasoning behind such analytical processes, even including instances where researchers went along with their instinctive hunches. Again, transparency is crucial as it enables the reader to pass better judgements on the analytical process and any conclusions drawn.

Is sufficient original material provided?

Any recurring themes identified by researchers in the analytical process should ideally be supported, where appropriate, by the inclusion of original material, such as excerpts, quotations, response series, numerical data, summaries, etc. These inclusions serve to corroborate any conclusions made by authors whilst also providing readers with an opportunity to make up their own minds (remember the subjective reality concept, p. 64).

Have the researchers been open about their own views?

The theoretical standpoint of the researchers conducting a qualitative study should be expressed freely and without reservation if readers are to be able to assess data accurately. The naturalistic concept of a subjective reality subscribed to by qualitative methods implies that the subjective perspective of a researcher cannot but influence the very nature of the data collected by them.

The researcher in a qualitative study is therefore regarded as an integral component of the research process, an instrument that inevitably influences the nature of data that can be gathered in a study. This effect is most profound with observational studies.

Are the efforts made to assess reliability stated?

The extent to which the identification of themes and the drawing of conclusions are consistent between researchers should be determined and stated in the study report. Ideally, more than one researcher should perform analysis of qualitative data. Even in studies performed by a single researcher, data should be presented to other colleagues for perusal in order to establish the reliability of the descriptions, interpretations and conclusions made by any one researcher.

Are the efforts made to establish validity of conclusions stated?

Authors should state any efforts made during the research process to increase the diversity and robustness of the collected data as well as efforts made to challenge the conclusions suggested by the data observations. Such a process can only increase the validity of qualitative result findings and the extent to which result findings can be generalized.

Strategies may include:

- Selection of further cases that can provide alternative or contradictory views to the mainstream obtained in a study.
- Selection of cases from opposing pressure groups.
- Use of different data collection methods.
- Selection of cases from different subsets of a population such as different ethnic groups.

How do the results affect the care of my patients?

In order to determine the applicability of qualitative results to the care of individual patients, questions that need to be asked should include:

- Whether the issues addressed were those that concern your patients?
- How applicable are the issues raised to your patients' socio-cultural or religious beliefs?
- Whether raised issues could confer any added benefit to your patients?
- What are your patients' feelings about the issues raised in the qualitative study?
- Are the involved subjects from the study too dissimilar from your patients?

This is where your clinical judgement based on experience and expertise comes in yet again.

Glossary of terms

Incidence Number of new cases arising over a specified time period.

Incidence rate Number of new cases in a defined population arising over a given time period.

Incidence proportion Proportion of the unaffected 'at risk' individuals in a defined population who will contract the disease of interest over a given period.

Prevalence Total number of existing cases of a disease in a defined population over a stated period.

Prevalence rate Proportion of a defined population with a disease over a time period.

Point prevalence Proportion of a defined population known to have a disease at a particular point in time.

Period prevalence Proportion of the population recorded as having a disease over a specified period.

Standardized mortality ratio Ratio of actual deaths to expected deaths from a given condition or event. Useful for monitoring trends or changes in mortality rates associated with a particular condition by comparing observed death rates in a particular population with expected rates as observed in a standard population.

Reliability Reliability describes the consistency of test results on repeat measurements. Reliability values are expressed by correlation coefficients which range from 0.0 (*no agreement*) to 1.0 (*complete agreement*).

Correlation coefficients used in estimating reliability values include:

- Cronbach's alpha: used with complex tests comprising several sections or measuring several variables (e.g. the IQ test).
- Kappa statistic: used with tests measuring categorical variables (e.g. the driving test *vis-à-vis* safe driver/unsafe driver).
- Intraclass correlation coefficient (ICC): used with tests measuring quantitative variables (e.g. serum calcium).

Inter-rater reliability Describes the extent of agreement of test results when two or more assessors make simultaneous measurements, for example agreement between judges in gymnastic sporting events.

Test–retest reliability Describes the extent of agreement of initial test results with results of repeat measurement made later on.

Alternate-forms reliability Describes the extent of agreement of results when two similar types of tests make measurements of the same variable at the same time.

Split-half reliability Describes the extent of agreement of the results from two stable halves of a split test.

Validity The validity of a test describes the extent to which a test actually measures what it purports to measure.

Face validity This describes the extent to which a test appears to be measuring what it purports to measure, on inspection. Face validity is a weak type of validity because it is based on subjective judgements.

External validity This describes the extent to which results from a study can be generalized to a wider population.

Internal validity This describes the extent to which results from a study can be said to reflect the 'true' results when study design and methodology are taken into consideration. In other words, the extent to which test methodology permits reflection of the 'true picture'.

Content validity This describes the extent to which the variables or items (e.g. temperature) being measured by a test (e.g. thermometer) are related to that which should be measured by such a test.

Predictive validity This describes the extent to which a test result (e.g. positive pregnancy test) predicts what it should be logically expected to predict (i.e. cyesis). In other words, how accurately does a test predict the events we would expect from such test results?

Concurrent validity This describes the extent to which a test (e.g. driving test) distinguishes between the different samples it should be expected to distinguish between (e.g. safe driver/unsafe driver). This is usually determined by comparing the test with an external gold standard.

Criterion validity An umbrella term used in epidemiology encompassing predictive, concurrent, convergent and discriminant validity.

Cross-validity Describes the stability of a test's validity when applied to different subgroups of a target population.

Incremental validity Incremental validity compares a test with other related tests regarding the best reflection of a measured property.

Convergent validity Convergent validity describes the extent of correlation between results from a test with results obtained from other similar tests, that is, when applied simultaneously, similar tests measuring the same variables ought to show a correlation in their respective results.

Discriminant validity Discriminant validity describes the extent to which the results of a test are dissimilar from the results of another unrelated test, that is, when applied simultaneously, dissimilar tests that do not measure similar properties should not show a correlation in their respective results.

References and suggested further reading

Altman D. *Practical statistics for medical research*. London: Chapman & Hall, 1995.

Anderson B. *Methodological errors in medical research*. Oxford: Blackwell, 1990.

Antman EM, Lau J, Kupelnick B et al. A comparison of results of meta-analyses of randomized clinical trials and recommendations of clinical experts. *JAMA* 1992; **268**: 240–8.

Bero L, Rennie D. The Cochrane Collaboration: preparing, maintaining and disseminating systematic reviews of the effects of healthcare. *JAMA* 1995; **274**: 1935–8.

Bland M. *An introduction to medical statistics*. Oxford: Oxford University Press, 1987.

Bland M. *An introduction to medical statistics*. New York, NY: Oxford University Press, 1995.

Brown T, Wilkinson G. *Critical reviews in psychiatry*. College seminar series. London: Royal College of Psychiatrists, 1998.

Bush B, Shaw S, Cleary P et al. Screening for alcohol abuse using the CAGE questionnaire. *Am J Med* 1987; **82**: 231–6.

Campbell MJ, Machin D. *Medical statistics: a common sense approach*. Chichester: Wiley, 1999.

Cantona WJ, Hudson MA, Scardino PT et al. Selection of optimal prostatic specific antigen cut-offs for early diagnosis of prostate cancer: receiver operating characteristic curve. *J Urol* 1994; **152**: 2037–42.

Cartwright A. *Health surveys in practice and potential*. London: Kings Fund Publishing, 1983.

Chalmers TC, Celano P, Sacks HS et al. Bias in treatment assignment in controlled clinical trials. *N Eng J Med* 1983; **309**: 1358–61.

Colditz GA, Miller JA, Mosteller JF. How study design affects outcome in comparisons of therapy. I. Medical. *Stat Med* 1989; **8**: 441–54.

Collett D. *Modelling survival data in medical research*. London: Chapman & Hall, 1994.

Curran S, Williams CJ. *Clinical research in psychiatry – a practical guide*. Oxford: Butterworth-Heinemann, 1999.

Dixon R, Munroe J, Silcocks P et al. *The evidence-based medicine workbook: critical appraisal for clinical problem solving*. Oxford: Butterworth-Heinemann, 1997.

DoH (Department of Health). *Research and development: towards an evidence-based health*. London: HMSO, 1996.

Drummond MF, Maynard A. *Purchasing and providing cost effective healthcare*. Edinburgh: Churchill-Livingstone, 1993.

Drummond MF, O'Brien B, Stoddard GL, Torrance GW. *Methods for the economic evaluation of healthcare programmes* (second edition). Oxford: Oxford University Press, 1997.

Egger M, Smith G. Misleading meta-analysis. *BMJ* 1995; **311**: 753–4.

Elwood J. *Critical appraisal of epidemiological studies and clinical trials*. Oxford: Oxford University Press, 1998.

Fagan TJ. Nomogram for Bayes' theorem. *N Engl J Med* 1975; **293**: 257–61.

Farmer R, Miller D, Lawrenson R et al. *Lecture notes on epidemiology and public health medicine*. Oxford: Blackwell, 1996.

Gardner MJ, Altman DG. *Statistics with confidence: confidence intervals and statistical guidelines*. London: BMJ Publishing, 1989.

Gelder M, Gath D, Mayou R, Cowen P. *Oxford textbook of psychiatry*. Oxford: Oxford University Press, 1996.

Greenhalgh T. *How to read a paper: the basics of evidence-based medicine*. London: BMJ Publishing Group, 1997.

Greenhalgh T, Taylor R et al. How to read a paper: papers that go beyond numbers. (Qualitative research.) *BMJ* 1997; **315**: 740–3.

Grol R. Beliefs and evidence in changing clinical practice. *BMJ* 1997; **315**: 418–21.

Guyyatt G, Rennie D. Users' guides to medical literature. *JAMA* 1993; **270**: 2096–7.

Guyyatt GH, Sackett DL, Cook DJ. Users' guides to medical literature. II. How to use an article about therapy or prevention. A. Are the results of the study valid? *JAMA* 1993; **270**: 2598–601.

Guyyatt GH, Sackett DL, Cook DJ. Users' guides to medical literature. II. How to use an article about therapy or prevention. B. What were the results and will they help me in caring for my patients? *JAMA* 1994; **271**: 59–6301.

Jaeschke R, Guyyatt G, Sackett DL. Users' guides to medical literature. III. How to use an article about a diagnostic test. A. Are the results of the study valid? *JAMA* 1994; **271**: 389–91.

Jaeschke R, Guyyatt G, Sackett DL. Users' guides to medical literature. III. How to use an article about a diagnostic test. B. What were the results and will they help me in caring for my patients? *JAMA* 1994; **271**: 703–7.

Jefferson T, Demicheli V, Mugford M. *Elementary economic evaluation in healthcare*. London: BMJ Publishing Group, 1996.

Marmot M, Brunner E et al. Alcohol and cardiovascular disease: the status of the U-shaped curve. *BMJ* 1991; **303**: 565–8.

Moon G, Gould M et al. *Epidemiology – an introduction*. Buckingham: Open University Press, 2000.

O'Brien BJ, Heyland D, Richardson WS et al. Users' guides to medical literature. XIII. How to use an article on economic analysis of clinical practice. A. Are the results of the study valid? *JAMA* 1997; **227**: 1552–7.

O'Brien BJ, Heyland D, Richardson WS et al. Users' guides to medical literature. XIII. How to use an article on economic analysis of clinical practice. B. Are the results of the study valid? *JAMA* 1997; **227**: 1802–6.

Parmar MKB, Machin D. *Survival analysis, a practical approach*. Chichester: Wiley, 1995.

Pope C, Mays N. *Qualitative research in health care*. London: BMJ Publishing Group, 1999.

Puri BK, Hall AD. *Revision notes in psychiatry*. London: Arnold Publishers, 1998.

Rose G, Barker D. *Epidemiology for the uninitiated* (second edition). London: BMJ Publishing Group, 1986.

Sackett DL, Haynes RB, Tugwell P et al. *Clinical epidemiology – a basic science for clinical medicine* (second edition). Boston, MA: Little, Brown & Co., 1991.

Sackett DL, Richardson WS, Rosenberg WMC, Haynes RB. *Evidence-based medicine: how to practise and teach EBM*. Edinburgh: Churchill-Livingstone, 1997.

Staus S, Sackett D. Using research findings in clinical practice. *BMJ* 1998; **317**: 339–42.

Streiner DL, Norman GR. *Health measurement scales*. Oxford: Oxford Medical University Press, 1989.

Swinscow TDV. *Statistics at square one*. London: BMJ Publishing Group, 1996.

Temple RJ. A regulatory authority's opinion about surrogate endpoints. In: Nimmo WS, Tucker GT, eds. *Clinical measurement in drug evaluation*. New York, NY: J Wiley, 1995.

Index